SWITCHOVER!

OTHER KEATS COOKBOOKS

ADD A FEW SPROUTS
by Martha H. Oliver

BETTER FOOD FOR BETTER BABIES
by Gena Larson

BIRCHER-BENNER CHILDREN'S DIET BOOK

BIRCHER-BENNER RAW FRUITS AND VEGETABLES BOOK

COOKING WITH VITAMINS
by Martha H. Oliver

EVERYBODY'S FAVORITE (ORTHOMOLECULAR) MUFFIN BOOK
by Rose Hoffer and Muriel Warrington

GOOD FOOD, GLUTEN FREE
by Hilda Cherry Hills

GOOD FOOD, MILK-FREE, GRAIN-FREE
by Childa Cherry Hills

GOOD FOOD TO FIGHT MIGRAINE
by Hilda Cherry Hills

GOOD FOODS THAT GO TOGETHER
by Esther L. Smith

NATURAL FOODS BLENDER COOKBOOK
by Frieda Nusz

REAL FOOD COOKBOOK
by Ethel Renwick

SUPER SOY!
by Barbara Farr

TILDA'S TREAT
by Karen Kelly and Joan Hopkins

TOTAL VEGETARIAN COOKING
by Nathaniel Altman

WAY WITH HERBS COOKBOOK
by Bonnie Fisher

WHOLE-GRAIN BAKING SAMPLER
by Beatrice Trum Hunter

YOGURT, KEFIR AND OTHER CULTURES
by Beatrice Trum Hunter

SWITCHOVER!

The Anti-Cancer Cooking Plan For Today's Parents and Their Children

RUTH YALE LONG, Ph.D.

KEATS PUBLISHING, INC. NEW CANAAN, CONNECTICUT

Library of Congress Cataloging in Publication Data

Long, Ruth Yale.
  Switchover! : the anti-cancer cooking plan for today's parents and their children.

  Bibliography: p.
  Includes index.
  1. Cancer—Nutritional aspects. 2. Cancer—Diet therapy—Recipes.
I. Title.
RC263.L65 1984   641.5′63   84-16386
ISBN 0-87983-400-5 (pbk.)

SWITCHOVER!
The Anti-Cancer Cooking Plan for Today's Parents and Their Children

Keats edition published 1984 by Keats Publishing, Inc.
Copyright © 1983 by Ruth Yale Long, Ph.D.
Originally published by Nutrition Education Association, Inc., Houston, Texas.
Reprinted by arrangement with the author.

ISBN: 0-87983-400-5

Printed in the United States of America

Keats Publishing, Inc.
27 Pine Street (Box 876)
New Canaan, Connecticut 06840

CONTENTS

INTRODUCTION

We can help prevent cancer and other infectious and degenerative diseases if we eat good, natural food. If every cell in our body gets every nutrient it needs, every cell, every tissue and every organ will be healthy and *we'll* be healthy.

That may sound too simple, but it's true. I believe everyone would agree that if every cell in his own liver were healthy, his liver would be healthy. It's true of every other tissue and organ as well.

A normal, healthy cell will never turn into a cancer cell. It must be deprived of oxygen or of some other nutrient before the change to cancer, arthritis, digestive problems, Alzheimer's or any other disease will develop. Infectious diseases are included in this list because if every cell in the immune system is healthy, it will protect us from colds, flu, pneumonia and even cancer.

Most cancer researchers realize that all of us have precancerous cells that develop from cells damaged by X-rays, injury or poor food, but if our immune system is healthy, it will destroy the precancerous cells before they can develop into cancer.

Many health-related organizations are now emphasizing the importance of diet for prevention and control of cancer and other diseases. The American Cancer Society has published suggestions for cancer prevention. Dr. Frank J. Rauscher Jr., Vice-President for Research of the Society, suggests that we adopt the following measures:

1. Reduce total fats, both saturated and unsaturated, by 25 percent.

2. Eat plenty of fruits, vegetables and whole-grain cereal products, especially those high in vitamin C and in beta-carotene, which the body changes to vitamin A. Particularly recommended are oranges, grapefruit, dark green leafy vegetables, carrots, winter squash, tomatoes, beans, nuts, seeds, and vegetables in the cabbage family.

3. Reduce our intake of salt-cured, salt-pickled and smoked foods.

4. The Society says we can drink alcoholic beverages moderately, but let's avoid them altogether, except maybe a little wine with dinner on special occasions.

Dr. Rauscher believes that the many treatments now being used in what he calls the "golden age of cancer treatment" can bring an end to "the threat of the disease by the end of the century, if not sooner." What a tremendous boon to mankind, that *if we want to,* we can help prevent our own cancers and other diseases.

The American Cancer Society is not a voice crying in the wilderness. Nutritionists have emphasized the importance of food for many years. Dr. George Blackburn, a Harvard surgeon, says that cancer patients might respond better to treatment if they were better nourished. Dr. Paul Marks of Columbia University College of Physicians and Surgeons says that as many as one-half of fatal cancers in women and one-third in men may be attributed in part to diet. Dr. Michael B. Sporn of the National Cancer Institute notes that more than half of all human cancers start in skin tissue inside or outside the body. Since all skin cells depend on vitamin A to develop normally, the vitamin helps defend the body against cancer and even helps keep cancer cells from forming.

Dr. Harry B. Demopoulos of the New York University Medical Center says that 80 percent of all human cancer is environmental;

however, less than 1 percent of cancers are caused by industrial chemicals. The rest are caused by our internal environment, which is damaged by alcohol, by smoking and especially by the poor food we eat.

We know now that we are not helpless against the scourge of cancer. We can be responsible for our own health, and we can choose to eat well and prevent cancer from touching us and our families. Most people have not heard that more children age one to fourteen die of cancer than of any other disease. The time to change to natural food is now.

It is easy to switch over to natural foods. The food plan that you have in your hands consists of a moderate amount of protein, a small amount of fat and a lot of complex carbohydrates, but not one bit of white sugar, white flour or white rice. We should eat moderate amounts of fish, legumes (beans, peas and peanuts), and whole fruits (no fruit juice, it's too sweet); rather large amounts of vegetables, both steamed and raw, and whole grains; and small amounts of yogurt, natural light-colored cheese, nuts and seeds; chicken from health food stores and one or two eggs a day, also from health food stores or from a farmer who raises chickens for his own family.

Red muscle meat (steaks, roasts, chops, and hamburger) and milk are best eaten sparingly or not at all. Cancer patients should probably eat no animal protein while their cancer is active.

We won't gain weight on this program because the food is so satisfying, we won't overeat. Many people have told me they could finally stop smoking when they eat this way because they no longer crave cigarettes.

The *Switchover* food plan is quick, easy, delicious and nutritious. There are many quick tricks in this book, because no one wants to stay in the kitchen all day. You'll never get tired of preparing food, and you'll never get bored eating it. The variety is tremendous. I have a lot of fun using different combinations of food and trying out new recipes. If you haven't eaten millet, cous-cous, homemade pizza, carob clusters, or vegetables lightly steamed in butter, you have a treat in store.

HOW TO USE THIS BOOK

The best way to start with this book is to read it all the way through, or at least scan it. Then go back to page 18 and make out your shopping list. On page 20 you'll find suggestions for preparing foods ahead, and also beginning on page 20 are the menus for each day for two weeks.

You'll notice that we suggest whole fruit for between-meal snacks, with vegetables for lunch and supper. That isn't a hard and fast rule. This diet is so flexible that you can have cottage cheese for breakfast and have your eggs in salad at noon—whatever is convenient. But if you follow the suggestions, you will be getting all the nutrients you need from all the different foods and you won't forget anything or miss getting a good variety of healthful foods.

Now you're off and running. You're headed for a new way of life. Please let me know if you have any suggestions for the next edition of this book. You may write to me at P.O. Box 20301, Houston, TX 77225.

Cordially,
RUTH YALE LONG, Ph.D.

1

CANCER AND NUTRITION RESEARCH

The story of nutrition and cancer is a promising one. It is the story of years of little-known research to prevent and control cancer.

This chapter explains the research on cancer pertaining to the immune system, proteins, carbohydrates, fats, fiber, obesity and the influence of microorganisms in the intestines.

If our cells get every nutrient they need in sufficient amounts, the cells will not change to cancer cells. Many modern nutritionists have accepted this idea for years, and many scientific researchers realize it's true.

There are several new terms now being used in discussing nutritional prevention of cancer (Jansson, 1978): "anticarcinogen," for example. A carcinogen is something that causes cancer. An anticarcinogen is something that keeps the carcinogen from causing cancer. Anticarcinogens are nutrients such as vitamin A, vitamin C, selenium (a mineral) and most of the other fifty or more nutrients.

Other new terms are "chemo-prevention" and "chemo-protection." Let's emphasize the "prevention" and "protection" aspects of these terms. Thus, "chemo-protection" means supplying the cells with enough vitamin A and all other nutrients to make sure they are healthy.

DIET AND CANCER

A panel of nutrition-minded scientists reported to Congress in 1976 (Houston *Chronicle*) that the diet should include less fat, less meat, less sugar and starch and more fruits and vegetables, with no smoking and very little alcohol. Exercise is important. Dr. Paul Marks of Columbia University was quoted as saying,

"As many as half of fatal cancers in women and one-third in men may be attributed in part to diet." Did you go to your physician or nutritionist the next day and demand a diet that would prevent cancer? I'm sure very few people, if any, did. We should have.

After that announcement, interest died down, and nothing much was mentioned in the news media about cancer and nutrition until June, 1982. The same exciting information as before was reported in newspapers, magazines, and on radio and TV, as the result of a study conducted by the National Academy of Sciences. The report urged Americans to cut down on alcohol, salt, fat and smoked foods, and eat more fruit, vegetables and whole grains. This is fundamentally what natural-food nutritionists have been saying for years, and it is what this book advocates. However, we will go much further into the details about what to eat and why.

The report says that the food we eat could be responsible for up to 40 percent of cancer in men and 70 percent in women (even higher than the previous report). Dr. Clifford Grobstein, an experimental biologist at the University of California at San Diego, and chairman of the study, said that damage to the body caused by eating poor food may be reversed if we eat better, more nutritious food, which is natural food—unrefined and unprocessed.

The report lists several guidelines for a better diet:
1. Cut down the consumption of fats, both saturated and unsaturated, to a total of 30 percent of calories. It is now more than 40 percent. (I have asked top nutritionists if less would be

better—for example, 20 percent of calories. They answered, "Oh, of course, but you might not get people to change their diets that drastically. We have to bring about the change gradually." I say change now before it's too late.) Fat is more closely related to cancers of the breasts, prostate, large bowel and some other cancers than any other food.

2. Cut out salt-cured, salt-pickled and smoked foods. People in Japan, China and Iceland have higher rates of esophagus and stomach cancer than people in other areas, and they eat high amounts of these foods.

3. We should stop smoking and drinking. (This is well known, and most cancer patients do stop. However, it is a little late by then. Let's stop now, before cancer strikes.)

4. Avoid exposure to molds, bacteria, pesticide residues and food additives that might be carcinogenic.

5. Guard against anything that can cause a cell mutation, such as oils that have been depigmented, deodorized, or hydrogenated (margarine and hard white shortening) as well as bottled oils, whether cold pressed or not. Rancidity in these oils damages cells. Avoid X-rays unless absolutely essential. Avoid drugs, even if prescribed by a doctor, if at all possible. A natural food diet will usually keep us healthy without drugs. Obviously, avoid hard drugs or over-the-counter drugs. All of these substances can cause damage to cells, which may lead to cancer. A normal healthy cell can never turn into a cancer cell.

THE IMMUNE SYSTEM

A great deal of research on the immune system shows its importance in preventing and controlling cancer. Let's find out how the immune system works, because if it is weak and your diet poor, and you have already been diagnosed as having cancer, the first thing to do is to build up your immune system. What do we mean by "the immune system" and how does it work?

The immune system uses several kinds of white blood cells to fight bacteria, viruses, and cancer cells in the body (Huemer, 1976). The first of the white blood cells are called polys, short for polymorphonuclear lymphocytes, which means cells with many forms of the nucleus. These cells have three or more lobes in their nucleus, which allow them to squeeze into very small places to get at the viruses. If the nucleus were large, the white cell could not squeeze through small openings. But each nucleus is shaped like a series of balloons that do not have much air in them. Thus, the balloons can be pulled through a small opening a little at a time until the entire balloon is on the inside of the virus.

HOW IT WORKS

When the polys meet the first microbes, millions of the white cells and of the bacteria are killed. The dead polys become pus, which means that they have done their work and the infection is over, but the sick person is still alive and getting better.

Other white cells are called macrophages—big eaters. They eat filth, whether it's spoiled food, damaged and dead cells, live and dead bacteria or any other garbage that needs to be cleaned up.

There are several different kinds of lymphocytes—defense cells from the lymph system. T cells (named for the thymus gland where they are made) patrol the area and fight one to one. They can quickly kill cancer cells. The theory is that T cells are the first line of defense against cancer.

Also in the category of lymphocytes are B cells, which get their name because they are made in the bone marrow. They use chemicals in their fight—antibodies which are proteins that attach themselves to foreign invaders such as allergens, bacteria, viruses and others. If there are plenty of antibodies, and if they are strong enough to attack and attach themselves to the invaders, the invaders don't have a chance to win the battle. Our antibodies will win and protect us from cancer.

But the number of antibodies we make depends partly on the amount of hydrochloric acid (HCl) we have in our stomachs to change the protein we eat to amino acids, which are the critical ingredients in the manufacture of antibodies. If we have only nineteen amino acids ready to make an antibody that requires twenty for its manufacture, we don't make nineteen-twentieths of the antibody; we can't make any of it. Thus, many of us can't fight the cancer cells because we don't have the number and amount of amino acids needed.

How do we get enough hydrochloric acid to make amino acids? By eating natural foods with plenty of protein from plants—whole grains and legumes (beans and peas). We also need complex carbohydrates (vegetables and whole fruits), natural animal fats (butter) and natural vegetable fats (nuts and seeds).

Of great importance to our supply of hydrochloric acid is not to drink water or other beverages with meals. We drink water thirty minutes before meals so the water can go through the stomach into the small intestine and leave the stomach free from anything that would dilute the hydrochloric acid.

We eat no white flour or white sugar or anything made from those nonfoods. We eat no cereal from supermarkets—we buy it all from health food stores, but we don't buy processed cereals there, either. We make all our own bread, biscuits, and muffins.

Also, the more sugar we eat, the more likely we are to have low blood sugar because the more sugar in our blood, the more insulin is secreted by the pancreas; insulin takes sugar out of the blood, and our blood sugar goes down. Low blood sugar is a forerunner of many diseases because it damages cells by not allowing them to make the energy they need for their many functions. Also, when the blood is full of sugar, the white blood cells don't work. They can be seen under a microscope, but they just sit there—they don't do their share as part of the immune system.

Let's use a sinus allergy as an example of how the immune system works. When there is a lot of pollen in the air, the pollen gets into the sinus cavities. If the cells that line the cavity are healthy and moist, the pollen slides out of the sinuses into the throat, down into the stomach and intestines and out of the body. That person doesn't have an allergic reaction. But if the sinus cells aren't moist, the pollen burrows into the dry sinus cavity, and the body goes into action to reject the pollen. First, fluid filled with histamine surrounds the pollen and walls it off so it can't spread through the bloodstream and affect other cells. Next, the adrenal glands pour out hormones which make antibodies that go through the blood and surround the pollen and other allergens and destroy them.

Histamine is good at first to wall off the allergen. But when it returns to the blood and travels through the bloodstream into the liver, histamine should be destroyed by an enzyme called histaminase. If the liver isn't healthy, it can't make histaminase, and the histamine keeps circulating and irritating tissues. You may know people who have to buy antihistamines because their own livers can't make the histaminase they need.

This entire process is called the inflammatory reaction. It goes to work when a precancerous cell is in the blood, and it destroys the cell before cancer can become established. The inflammatory process is known to be essential to health and to destroying the cancer. Many researchers are working on ways to strengthen the immune system so cancer won't develop.

What can strengthen the immune system? All protective nutrients, especially proteins, are needed. All cells that are damaged by nutritional deficiencies or injury must be immediately repaired or the damaged cell may turn into a cancer cell. As we've said, a normal. healthy cell will never turn into a cancer cell. Easily assimilated proteins such as free amino acids are helpful, plus plant proteins, which can be digested with the help of digestive enzymes. Massive amounts of vitamin C and vitamin A are required. All other nutrients must be available for the body to use as needed. With a complete arsenal of nutrients, the immune system can prevent or fight cancer.

VITAMINS

All the vitamins help the immune system work. Vitamin A helps, first, to stimulate the production of antibodies, to protect against powerful bacteria and to keep the immune system from being suppressed by cortisone.

B vitamins are co-enzymes, so they are needed to help manufacture antibodies. All other vitamins and minerals are needed as well. There is no one magic pill that will, all by itself, keep the entire immune system working.

Vitamin C has a lot to do with this battle plan. It seems to kill viruses and to entice the macrophages to eat more garbage. It helps build up the cells, and it also assists in the manufacture of complement, a substance which helps the antibodies work.

Vitamin E helps produce more antibodies than are possible otherwise. It has many other uses. It is an antioxidant, which means that it keeps oxygen from being used up quickly. Thus we have more oxygen, which is required for metabolism (use of foods). All of our cells eat and breathe, and vitamin E helps them breathe. It also helps pick up poisons, especially minerals such as lead and mercury, and get rid of them. These poisons damage cells and set up a climate that leads to cancer if we can't get enough vitamin E.

Vitamin E also helps keep vitamin A from being toxic. It helps fight foreign invaders. There are precautions with vitamin E. If you have high blood pressure, congestive heart failure, rheumatic fever or diabetes, start with small amounts and build up gradually.

It is now believed that if a pregnant woman doesn't get the nutrients she needs, her immune system will be weak, and she can pass the weakness on to her children, even to the second generation. Thus it is thought that some people who have frequent infections and later develop cancer had mothers who were malnourished during their pregnancy and after they were born. If there were not enough nutrients to make colostrum (the baby's defense against foreign invaders), there wouldn't be enough antibodies to keep the new baby well. Later, the baby loses its immunity from the colostrum and has to make its own antibodies. That's the reason babies are vaccinated against certain diseases. Their bodies can then make a lot of white blood cells which can react quickly against foreign invaders—bacteria, viruses or cancer cells.

When the immune system is activated by a vaccine, it can fight off the bacteria easily because the second time antibodies are called out, the response is quicker and more antibodies are made faster. The vaccine called BCG, which is used by many therapists, reacts on many fronts and can activate antibodies against cancer.

Immunity was "discovered" as a cancer treatment about fifteen years ago, but the importance of nutrition hasn't yet been accepted by most cancer physicians. As soon as the majority of physicians realizes the need for nutrients to keep the immune system working for us, that is how soon there will be a tremendous turnaround to success in the treatment of cancer.

You and I don't have to wait for the turnaround. We can prime our immune system with good food—beginning today.

PROTEINS

There seems to be much controversy over the amount of protein that cancer patients need. I believe that recent research helps us understand the problem. Most investigators say "no animal protein, at least for the first few months." Haenszel et al. (1973) agree that cancer of the colon has a higher correlation with a high beef intake than with any other food in the diet.

But Cheraskin et al. (1977) say that lack of protein in the diet can show up as cancer, especially in the liver and urinary tract. However, it is rare that protein is the only nutrient lacking—usually vitamins and minerals are also missing.

Protein from raw egg white was formerly thought to cancel out the good effects of the B vitamin biotin, but egg white protein has been found to reduce the incidence of liver cancer (Cheraskin, 1977).

A study was done with sixty-four terminal cancer patients who were suffering from severe ill health and malnutrition. Most were bedfast, and all were hospitalized. They were fed 210 mg of protein a day in a diet of 3,500 calories a day. The results were "truly remarkable." Most of the patients were near death when they entered the hospital, but after the food program, most of them could walk, they were more comfortable and they could take care of themselves. Many of them left the hospital and went home to live with their families.

In another study, patients who were force-fed diets containing 40 to 80 grams of protein a day gained strength, but when the feeding was stopped, their cells accumulated a great deal of water, and the cancers grew.

The answer to the controversy of too much or too little protein probably depends on how well the digestive system works. If it does not work well, the protein is not digested; it becomes a poison in the system, and it makes the disease worse.

However, if the protein is taken in the form of amino acids, which go quickly to the bloodstream and to the cells without having to be digested, tissue can be repaired, and the patient improves. There is a new interest among researchers in amino acids to help prevent, control or cure many diseases. A new era is opening in the use of these required nutrients. Amino acids are available now in health food stores. They should not be confused with protein powders or with predigested protein, which might have been changed to polypeptides but not to amino acids. The label should say "free" amino acids.

With amino acids, the patient's own digestive tract and all other cells can be repaired to help his body fight the cancer. Also, amino acids can be used to make enzymes that break down the tumor capsule, without the strain on the body of digesting the proteins to amino acids (Cheraskin, 1977).

REFINED CARBOHYDRATES

If we eat a lot of sugar, we are more likely to develop cancer, especially of the prostate, breast, ovaries, bladder, colon and rectum.

Excessive glucose helps cancer cells spread. But when complex carbohydrates from natural whole grains were given to experimental animals, the number of cases of cancer decreased (Shennan and Bishop, 1976).

Tumors must have sugar to thrive, so if it is possible to remove all or part of a large tumor surgically, the patient can survive more easily and fight the cancer better because the tumor is not there to use up the sugar, which the body needs in moderation for energy.

FATS AND OILS

Fats and oils have a high correlation with cancer, especially cancer of the colon. There are 92,500 new cases a year, with 47,400 deaths. The median survival time after discovery is 2.2 years (Shennan and Bishop, 1976).

Polyunsaturated fatty acids (PUFA) have been found to cause cancer because those fats become rancid in our bodies and damage cells. To prevent the damage, antioxidants such as vitamins A, C, and E, methionine (an amino acid) and selenium (a mineral) must be eaten in plentiful amounts. A study was reported in *Nutrition Today* (July–August, 1980) that showed that when people consumed more PUFA (supposedly to keep from having heart disease and strokes), there were just as many deaths from those illnesses, and there were even more deaths from cancer. Why? Because the oils damaged the cells, but no antioxidants were given to keep the damaged cells from becoming cancerous.

Another experiment with rats, some painted with coconut oil and some with corn oil, showed that more cancers of the liver were formed by the corn oil than by the coconut oil, which is a saturated fat (Clayson, 1975). It may be that the high intake of fat, with its damaging effects on the body, combined with deficiencies of the protective nutrients vitamin E and selenium, is related to cancers of the colon and breast.

Several types of skin cancer seem to be caused by large intakes of animal fats (Cheraskin, 1977). Also, if a patient eats more fat without increasing his intake of choline, he often develops a fatty liver, and the cancer spreads.

FIBER

If we eat enough fiber, we will eliminate body wastes quickly. Otherwise, the wastes stack up against the walls of the colon and cause sores which can turn into cancer. The best fiber seems to come from whole grains; next, from vegetables and whole fruits, all of which are often lacking in the average American diet. One of my favorite quotations is from Josef Issels, a cancer specialist in Germany. He said, "Whole grains are foods of incomparable perfection." I might add, refined grains are not just a "zero," they are actually a "minus." They damage cells by depriving them of needed nutrients.

OVERWEIGHT

People who are overweight past middle age are more likely to get cancer than people who are not. The major cancers they suffer from are cancers of the intestines, liver, gallbladder and genitourinary organs. Patients with endometrial cancer are often overweight, they have blood sugar problems, no children, and have had several abortions. Of overweight patients given radiation treatments for cancer of the cervix, only 38 percent who weighed over 170 pounds lived five years, but 55 percent who weighed less than 170 pounds survived five years.

If animals eat plenty of vitamins and minerals but less food, they have fewer cancers. This follows the nutrition plan in this book, which emphasizes the importance of eating small amounts of food six times a day, rather than three larger meals a day. We can digest food better if we eat less at a time. Undigested food leads to the accumulation of poisons in the body, especially in the colon, and 30 percent of American cancers are cancers of the colon (Cheraskin, 1977).

MICROORGANISMS

Bile acids combined with microorganisms in the large bowel cause lesions which may become cancerous. Many deaths from cancer are related to infections caused by such microorganisms, which send poisons through the blood to any cell in the body. At the same time, the immune system is depressed, often because of treatment of the cancer with radiation and chemotherapy.

If enough of the microorganisms are held in one spot, they can cause infection or other disease because they overwhelm the body's im-mune system. Symptoms of large bowel cancer are bleeding, changes in bowel habits, weight loss, abdominal pain, or a feeling of not having completely eliminated fecal matter. A pleasant way to eliminate poisonous microorganisms is to take lactobacillus acidophilus—live friendly bacteria.

COMBINATION OF NUTRIENTS

Rats were given all essential nutrients but were also given fewer calories than required for normal growth. This underfeeding resulted in smaller but healthier adult animals, and a 35 percent increase in longevity. Their immune systems worked better longer, and they didn't develop spontaneous tumors so fast (Yunis and Greenberg, 1974).

Another study showed that smoking and drinking alcohol kept people from eating good foods, especially fruits, vegetables and milk. The risk of developing cancer is twenty-five times greater for a heavy whiskey drinker than for a non-drinker (Wynder and Bross, 1961).

In Sweden, there were formerly many cases of Plummer-Vinson disease (difficulty in swallowing, inflammation of the tongue, enlarged spleen and withering of the upper part of the esophagus). This disease often precedes cancer of the intestinal tract. Many drugs and all other possible therapies were tried, but none helped until vitamin and iron supplements were used (Wynder and Bross, 1961).

Although many experiments we've discussed have shown good results with single nutrients, we see the best results with all nutrients. Several researchers and physicians have had outstanding success with this therapy. These investigators point out that cancer is a degenerative disease caused by nutritional deficiencies, usually triggered by carcinogens of various types. These include chemicals in air, food, water, industrial operations and most of all, microbes that get into the body. Investigators have named deficiencies of many of the fifty or more protective nutrients as cancer-causing conditions.

2

DIET AND SUPPLEMENTS TO PREVENT CANCER

The only sensible way to avoid cancer is to prevent it and it can be prevented if we start soon enough. "Starting soon" should mean that your grandparents ate well. Since we can't go back, let's make sure that we eat well beginning now.

Our food program is a way of life—not a crash diet to follow for a week, a month, or even a year till we feel good, then go back to our old way of eating. We will get sick again, because the Standard American Diet (SAD) of processed and refined foods causes illness in the first place.

You will recover from almost every ailment with this food program. Dr. Tom Spies, an early nutritionist, said, "If we just knew enough, we could cure all our ailments with food." Hippocrates said, "Food is our medicine, our medicine is food."

NUTRITION PHILOSOPHY

Our philosophy of nutrition is that if every cell in the body gets the nutrients it needs, every cell, every tissue, every organ, will be healthy, and *we* will be healthy. Our food program is non-specific; which means that all ailments respond to it because all cells *need* all nutrients, and when they *get* all nutrients, all cells will be healthy. Therefore, when all nutrients get into the bloodstream, the nutrients will go to your scalp and cure dandruff, to your toes and cure athlete's foot, and to all the cells in between.

There is no other way to be well. All drugs have adverse reactions; all antibiotics damage the liver.

It is completely logical that food will keep us well. We were all once one cell. That cell had to have nutrients to divide and make more cells. Without division and, of course, multiplication, we would not have become the human beings we now are, with an average of 70 trillion cells.

Our cells are made of about fifty nutrients that they can't manufacture—about twenty vitamins, twenty minerals, eight amino acids (building blocks of protein), carbohydrates, fats and water. Each one of these nutrients is essential. "Essential" means that we would die without it.

We don't have to be sick. With good nutrition, we can be young, slim and energetic for years longer than we might think. This can be accomplished with a natural food diet—nothing highly processed. We allow other people to grind our whole grains into flour (owning a mill would be better so we can grind it ourselves—the flour is fresher), but we do the rest: we make our own bread, biscuits, crackers and pancakes.

SEVEN BASIC RULES FOR PREVENTION

Seven special rules guide our nutrition program to prevent cancer.

RULE 1: EAT SMALL MEALS

We eat six meals a day, three at regular meal times, and three snacks in between. We digest our food better if we eat small amounts more often. We used to have a saying, "We are what we eat." Now our saying is, "We are what we assimilate." The food must go to our blood in the proper form to nourish our cells. If we eat too much at one time, we overload our digestive system, and we don't have enough enzymes to break down the food to the forms that can go into the blood.

What are enzymes? They are substances that make reactions happen fast. The food would eventually break down even without enzymes, but it would take so long that we couldn't maintain health. Enzymes can break down (and build up) the forms of the food we need quickly. Food that goes into the blood undigested because enzymes are missing can cause disease anywhere in the body.

RULE 2: DON'T DRINK LIQUIDS WITH MEALS

We drink water at specified times—thirty minutes before our three meals and three snacks so the water will go through the stomach into the small intestine before the food gets to the stomach. Thus the stomach is free from anything that would dilute the hydrochloric acid it manufactures. The acid must be very strong to begin digesting protein, which is the one food that gets partially digested in the stomach.

We *never* drink coffee, tea, cola, cocoa, bottled drinks, canned drinks, alcohol or fruit juice. Fruit juice is too sweet, even if no sugar has been added. A glass of fruit juice has from four to seven teaspoons of sugar. Although the sugar is natural, it is too concentrated. Many people start their downfall to poor health by drinking a lot of fruit juice and causing their blood sugar to be low. It seems that eating sugar would cause blood sugar to be high, but the sugar makes the pancreas overreact and produce too much insulin, which then takes so much sugar out of the blood that we have low blood sugar. We eat whole, fresh, raw, ripe fruit. If we wish, we can drink organically grown vegetable juice.

Since all those beverages are prohibited, what does that leave us to drink? Milk and water. We can drink one glass of milk and one of yogurt if we insist, but none is required. Some nutritionists say adults shouldn't drink milk at all. The way milk is processed, much of the food value is destroyed.

Half the milk we drink should be yogurt, which is partially digested by the bacteria which make it sour. Yogurt is good to take our food supplement tablets with during meals because yogurt is thick, and the tablets go down easily.

That leaves water. We drink water thirty minutes before meals or two hours after. Since we eat about every two and one-half hours, two hours after a meal is the same time as thirty minutes before.

If you've ever had problems with gas, bloating or a too-full feeling after meals, this one small hint about not drinking liquids with meals might solve your digestive problems. If you haven't had any problems yet, do this to avoid future problems. Taking antacids to relieve gas and bloating may relieve the pain but it may also cause digestive diseases.

Why is it so important that we do not dilute the hydrochloric acid? Because without acid, we cannot digest proteins, and the undigested proteins lead to cancer.

Here's how digestion works. We chew the protein and turn it into polypeptide chains. Digestive enzymes break the chains apart, and the individual peptides pass into the small intestine where different enzymes break them open and release the amino acids, which can then be built up into tissue—hair, eyes, skin, blood, bones, teeth, and muscles, plus hormones, enzymes and all other body proteins.

The HCl must be very strong. If you know about the pH scale, it is the scale used to measure acids and alkalines anywhere—in industry, in your garden and in your body. It runs from zero (very acid) to 14 (very alkaline). Our stomach acid is secreted at 0.8, which is very strong. By the time it gets mixed with the food we've eaten, the acid is diluted to 2 to 3 on the scale. That is exactly the right acidity to digest protein to peptides. But if we drink liquids with meals, we can dilute the acid to 4 to 5 on the pH scale. At that weak acidity, we cannot break the large protein molecules down to peptides (Guyton, 1976).

Therefore, our proteins go on into the small intestine, but there are not enough enzymes there to turn proteins into peptides—only enzymes that turn peptides into amino acids. So the undigested proteins continue through the twenty-five feet of small intestine, and collect in the sigmoid colon, way down low on the left side. The sigmoid colon is called that because it connects the descending colon on the left side with the rectum in the middle of the body by means of an "S" curve. "Sigmoid" is Greek for the letter "S."

The sigmoid colon is very muscular; it has to be to hold the fecal matter till it is time to send it to the rectum to be excreted. But everywhere there is a blood vessel that goes into the sigmoid to feed the colon itself, there is a little weak place. As the putrefying mass of undigested protein stays in the sigmoid, it causes tremendous gas pressure, which pushes putrefied fecal matter up beside the blood vessel at the weak place. It first makes a wedge shape, then continues to push up until it gets as big as a grape. The "grape" extends from the colon into the body cavity. The membrane that surrounds the "grape" is thin; it was formerly the thin membrane that lined the sigmoid colon. It has no muscles, so it can never push the putrefied fecal matter back into the colon. It stays there for life unless it is surgically removed. This "grape" is called a diverticulum; the illness is diverticulosis; and if there is inflammation the disease is called diverticulitis.

According to the *Journal of Diseases of the Colon and Rectum,* when people with these ailments are examined by their physicians, it is often impossible for the physician to know whether the disease is diverticulosis or cancer of the colon. The "grapes" cannot be removed even with a good diet of natural foods—there's no way to get rid of them except by surgery. Diverticulosis is often a forerunner of cancer of the colon, which is, as we've said, the second most common location of cancer in both men and women, right after cancer of the lung.

Even if you don't develop diverticulosis, poisonous bacteria in undigested protein can multiply and go into the bloodstream. They float along, and wherever they land, they can cause disease, including cancer, anywhere in the body.

You can tell if you have undigested protein stacking up in your colon; if your stools are dark colored and smell bad, you do. The stools should be light-colored, big around and soft, and have almost no odor. That means we have more friendly bacteria than poisonous bacteria in our intestines. Friendly bacteria help get rid of the poisons that may cause cancer and other diseases. Ninety-five percent of the bacteria in the colon will be friendly if the stools are as described. They will overpower the bad bacteria and keep us well, with a nice clean colon, and, most important, no constipation. This helps give us a healthy immune system. If we take lactobacillus acidophilus (not bulgaricus) we get good results quickly.

Many people as young as thirty do not make enough HCl. Studies show that most people make 12 percent less HCl at forty than they did at thirty. Thirty percent of people age sixty or more manufacture *no* HCl in their stomachs. They are very sick people.

What happens to those sixty-year-olds—and to all the people who, gradually through the years, lose their ability to assimilate food? Their health gradually deteriorates, and they suffer from fatigue, depression, arthritis, low and high blood sugar, heart problems, digestive problems, loss of teeth and even myasthenia gravis, multiple sclerosis, muscular dystrophy, cerebral palsy and cancer.

If we eat too much protein at a time, say a ten- or twelve-ounce steak, we probably don't have enough enzymes or enough HCl to digest it. That means more undigested protein to become poisonous and cause cancer. Also, if we don't eat *enough* protein, we won't make enough amino acids to repair tissue. Amino acids build and repair tissue all over the body, and without these building blocks of protein, if a cell is damaged, it will not be repaired. Any cell may be damaged by undigested proteins which can stack up in any cell like garbage. These damaged cells can turn into cancer cells.

After the food leaves the stomach, the peptides must be changed into amino acids with the help of enzymes manufactured in the pancreas. Also, carbohydrates and fats must be digested to their smallest parts—small enough to go through the bloodstream to every cell in the body to furnish energy for all the activities of the cells. Thus, if we don't manufacture enough bicarbonate or enzymes in the pancreas, we won't be able to digest proteins, carbohydrates and fats in the small intestine.

Just as I was writing this, a plea for funds for people with myasthenia gravis was aired on television. A ten-year-old child with MG told of her tragic illness, which could have been completely prevented with a good food and food supplement program. She had never been told that.

Thus, it isn't just the older people who lose their ability to digest food. At any age, if the acid in the stomach isn't being manufactured in plentiful amounts, and if the pancreas can't make bicarbonate and enzymes to digest carbohydrates and fats, even a child can develop a chronic degenerative disease.

Many of the people I counsel tell me that their doctors have said their diet isn't so bad, it just seems that they don't assimilate the food they eat.

That must be the most common complaint in the world, but every person who tells me that seems to think he or she is unique—that they're the only one who has the problem. Far from it. As we've seen, it is an almost universal complaint, but those people do not know *why* they aren't able to assimilate food.

Through the years of eating the Standard American Diet (SAD) of 30 percent white sugar and white flour products and 42 percent fat, disease develops. The other 28 percent or so is processed, canned, frozen vegetables and fruits—convenience foods—that have lost most of their food value in the processing.

It is not normal to be ill; yet illness is expected in our American culture. We go to doctors to get drugs to save our health, but our ailments are caused by nutritional deficiencies.

There is still another reason for the problem. If we don't have frequent bowel movements and let the wastes pass out of the body, they can react with bile salts and bad bacteria in the colon to cause lesions (sores). These sores may turn into cancer. A cancer starts from a damaged cell. Unrefined bran furnishes bulk, which will help us move our bowels more often. One to three teaspoons a day are suggested, more if needed, with plenty of water, because without water, bran and wastes can stop up the colon like a cork.

Sometimes people argue with me that they can't swallow food without water to wash it down. They are swallowing it whole; what they need to do is chew it longer. Others say our intestines need water to keep the food liquid

enough to be well churned and accessible to digestive enzymes. Our food plan includes vegetables and fruits at every meal and snack except breakfast. These foods are usually 90 percent water, which will allow plenty of liquid for digestion. Any more liquid can dilute the HCl too much. I get more letters from readers and from counselees telling the helpful response of their bodies to "no liquids with meals" than from any other one thing. Try it.

With all this at stake, let's summarize three important points:
1. don't drink liquids with meals;
2. don't take antacids; and
3. do take unrefined bran along with plenty of water before meals so you'll have two or three soft, well-formed bowel movements a day.

RULE 3: EAT RAW AND STEAMED VEGETABLES

The rest of the seven rules are much shorter. We eat raw vegetables and steamed vegetables every day.

The easiest way to get both kinds of vegetables into your day's meals is to eat salads at noon and steamed vegetables at the evening meal. It's easy to get a fairly good salad at a salad bar, restaurant or cafeteria. (However, the lettuce may be three weeks old and sprayed with formaldehyde or sulfites to make it appear fresh.) The best way to eat salads if you work or go to school is to take a brown bag lunch with washed and dried green leaves and other vegetables carried in a plastic bag and eaten with a few nuts and seeds rather than with a dressing made with salad oil.

If everyone in the family eats salads for lunch, they'll all be ready for steamed vegetables at dinner. A good steamer helps. Mine is a Wearever Rice Steamer. (Wearever doesn't pay me to say this.) It's good because it has no holes in the bottom of the steam pan; the condensation from the vegetables doesn't drop through the holes and get lost in the water below. The steam holes are around the top of the inner pan. I've recently found out that these steamers are no longer available. Maybe the company (or some other company) will start making them again if we all ask them to.

Another good thing about the steamer is that

it is wide and shallow. I have little pans in which I pack and freeze meal-size portions of cooked protein foods—bean and/or grain burgers or loaves, meat loaves, roast beef, millet souffle and others. I get them out of the freezer in the morning and leave them in the fridge all day.

I go into the kitchen thirty minutes before a meal, drink my water first, then load the steamer with the little pans of protein foods surrounded by vegetables, set the timer and go on about my business. When the timer goes off, dinner is ready. I haven't had to stir anything, and it can't burn! That's the easiest food preparation I know of.

RULE 4: VARY YOUR DIET

We vary our diets as much as possible. On the prevention diet, we can eat a small amount of yogurt every day and one or two eggs if we're not subject to infections. If we are, our immune system is not working well. We need a healthy immune system to handle possible dangerous microorganisms in eggs. Buy your eggs at the health food store. We vary our vegetables, fruits, legumes, whole grains, nuts, seeds and other proteins.

RULE 5: DON'T EAT WHITE SUGAR OR WHITE FLOUR

We don't eat white sugar, white flour, white rice or any product made from those non-foods. These are the worst of the junk foods. (To make brown sugar, see recipe on p. 109.)

RULE 6: DON'T EAT CANNED OR FROZEN FOODS

We don't eat convenience foods, processed and refined by someone else. We can freeze grains and legumes ourselves for future meals, and vegetables and fruits if we grow them in our own garden. We eat no more than four ounces of red meat (steaks, roasts, chops and hamburger) four times a week. We can eat calves' liver in addition. The calves' livers detoxify the poisons in their food, air and water,

but the poisons aren't stored in the liver—they're sent to the fat cells, which is one reason why we should cut down on red meat, especially well-marbled meat. Other reasons are that our digestive system is overworked by trying to digest eight-, ten- and twelve-ounce steaks, and our kidneys have trouble filtering the wastes from so much red meat.

Most important, we don't eat processed meats such as lunch ham, bacon, sausage or hot dogs, or processed cheese. We don't eat cheese with orange dyes; we eat natural, light colored cheese such as Swiss, jack and mozzarella.

While I was earning a master's degree in public health with a major in nutrition, I was taught that every fiftieth chicken that goes through the slaughterhouse line has cancer. (Virginia Livingston-Wheeler, a well-known nutrition-minded physician in San Diego, says that after years of research she believes it is possible that "almost 100 percent of chickens" have cancer [Livingston-Wheeler, 1984].) The cancerous portion is cut off, thrown in a vat, cooked down and fed to the next batch of chickens. Thus, we're eating cancerous flesh, growth hormone, pesticides and antibiotics. The chickens are fed so much growth hormone that a chicken that should mature in ten to twelve weeks now goes to market in six, and the farmer makes twice as much money. The farmers say they can cut their time down to three weeks. This information persuades me to buy chicken at the health food store. Since it tastes so much better, we know that it must have been raised better. But chicken may not be good enough even there. Dr. Livingston-Wheeler says health food store chickens may have dangerous microbes that may cause cancer. Thus, if you are often ill with colds or other infections or severe allergies, your immune system may not be working well, and you may not be able to destroy the microbes in chicken. If you can't, you might get cancer.

RULE 7: EAT NUTS AND SEEDS

We don't use bottled vegetable oils because they have been deodorized, depigmented and sometimes hydrogenated (treated with hydrogen, which makes them saturated instead of unsaturated), and heated to high temperatures, even if the label says "cold pressed." All of these processes change the good fats needed by our bodies from a molecule called "cis," which we need, to a molecule called "trans," which our bodies can't use. If we eat the French fried potatoes, we've eaten the trans fats. Where are they? They stack up anywhere in the body and damage cells. I read that fifty-six different brands of margarine have been tested and all were found to contain trans fats. So we eat butter.

We do need vegetable oils—polyunsaturated fats—so how do we get them? We eat nuts and seeds; from three to six small measures a day. A small measure of nuts and seeds is the equivalent of one teaspoon of oil: two teaspoons of sesame, sunflower or pumpkin seeds, two walnut halves, four pecan halves, six almonds or twelve peanuts. Vary these servings, and if you're a little lady, you'll probably need three servings; if a big man, six.

Sometimes people laugh and say, "Do you really count out twelve peanuts and eat just that many?" I usually just pick up a few, and if there are eleven or thirteen, that's near enough.

To review the prevention diet: we eat very little red meat, no supermarket chickens, small amounts of nuts and seeds, moderate amounts of cheese, one or two eggs a day from the health food store and lots of fish, whole grains combined with legumes (beans, peas and peanuts), fresh vegetables and whole fruits.

MEALS TO PREVENT CANCER

Let's paint a word picture of a day's intake of food to see how easily we can carry out our new food program.

On arising: drink water. No one can tell you how much to drink. You may need six, eight, ten or even twelve ounces. If you drink too much, you will be waterlogged, and you won't enjoy your breakfast; if you drink too little, you'll be constipated the next day.

BREAKFAST: 1 or 2 eggs, wholegrain cereal (biscuits, muffins, bread, crackers, pancakes, waffles); dry cereal (granola without sugar); or cooked cereal such as oatmeal or cracked wheat— all from the health food store.

Thirty minutes before snack: water.

MID-MORNING SNACK: whole raw, ripe fruit and protein. Choices may include a graham cracker you made plus peanut butter, natural light-colored hard cheese, cottage cheese, yogurt, mixed nuts and seeds.

Thirty minutes before lunch: water.

LUNCH: 4 to 6 ounces of a high-protein dish plus raw or steamed green or yellow vegetables, small amount of potato if you wish, unless you need to gain weight—then eat a large amount.

Thirty minutes before snack: water.

MID-AFTERNOON SNACK: Same as mid-morning; vary the fruit and protein.

Thirty minutes before dinner: water.

DINNER: Same as lunch; different vegetables, different protein.

Thirty minutes before snack: water.

EVENING SNACK: Same as mid-morning; vary the protein, vary the fruit.

EVERY DAY: Three to six small measures of nuts and seeds. Also every day, several times a day: whole grains that you made into bread, biscuits, crackers or muffins.

SPECIAL FOODS

The following special foods are well known for their health-giving qualities:

NUTRITIONAL OR FOOD YEAST: This is often called brewer's yeast because the first such yeast was a by-product of the brewing industry, and the old name is often used. We should eat nutritional or food yeast. Add to a drink made of milk or nut milk, raw egg and lecithin, flavored with any raw fruit, vanilla or nutmeg.

LIVER: Eat liver fresh or dried and powdered. Excellent food because of its high vitamin, mineral and protein content.

GARLIC: furnishes protection against pollution, heart disease, cancer, infections and especially high blood pressure. Take in perle or tablet form, up to three with each main meal.

LECITHIN: helps dissolve fatty deposits in the liver and arteries. Choose a brand with a high percentage of phosphatidyl choline and take according to the label.

UNREFINED BRAN: helps prevent constipation or diarrhea. Can be taken by the tablespoon in severe cases, always with plenty of water. Also add bran to all baked goods.

FOOD SUPPLEMENTS

How many vitamins and minerals should we take to prevent cancer, and other degenerative diseases, and why do we have to take them?

We can't get enough nutrients from food, even if we try, since most of it is sprayed, refined, processed and shipped long distances, all of which destroys much of the food value. So we take supplements—vitamins and minerals in tablet form—and other special foods.

I'll give amounts suggested for the average adult. Children age thirteen and up should take the adult dose; ages six to twelve, half that amount, and one to six, one-fourth that amount. Children up to one year old should be on breast milk or on a formula which includes brewer's yeast and vitamin C. Liquid vitamins are available from the health food store.

We take our tablets during a meal with yogurt. Hold a swallow of yogurt in your mouth, tilt your head back, drop a few tablets in your mouth (start with one) and swallow. The tablets go down easily with the thick liquid.

VITAMIN A: 25,000 IU, 1 or more a day of pro-vitamin A as beta-carotene, which is changed to vitamin A in the body when needed, or of fish liver oil.

VITAMIN B: B complex formula containing about 30 mg of B1, B2, and B6; 150 mg of B3 and pantothenic acid, plus all the rest of the Bs. Take 2 tablets a day to begin with, increase to 5 a day to determine the amount your own body needs for pep and energy, then after a few weeks or months, depending on your health, reduce to 2 a day for maintenance. B vitamins and C are needed in larger than usual amounts when we're under stress, so you may need to adjust your intake up or down as your stress level changes. Remember, cold weather is a stress on the body, as are extra work and play.

VITAMIN C: Take bowel tolerance of this vitamin. That means as much as you can take without getting gas or diarrhea. The amount will probably range between 1,000 and 10,000 mg a day.

VITAMIN D: 400 to 1,000 IU a day.

VITAMIN E: If you have diabetes, heart problems or high blood pressure, begin with 30 IU of vitamin E a day, increase by 30 IU a day every month, until at the end of a year you're taking 360 IU a day. If none of these conditions exist, young men can begin with 600 IU, young women with 400. By the time we're seventy, the suggested amount is 1,200 IU, so increase to the amount needed according to your age.

MINERALS: A multi-mineral tablet with about 1,000 mg of calcium, 500 mg of magnesium, 20 mg iron, 1 mg copper, 10 mg manganese, 200 mcg chromium, 225 mcg iodine, 22.5 mg zinc, 95 mg potassium and 200 mcg selenium is a well-balanced formula. If you can't find this formula, get the closest one to it and fill in with additional minerals bought individually.

LACTOBACILLUS ACIDOPHILUS (LA): These friendly bacteria live in our intestines and help destroy poisonous microorganisms. LA comes in tablet, powder and liquid form. Follow directions on the label.

These supplements are suggested for everyone every day from now on, because many of the vitamins and minerals are refined out of our food. Sick people may need more of many nutrients. For example, arthritics may need more calcium and magnesium. Amino acid chelated minerals are suggested.

Other supplements in tablet form that are helpful for many people are L-glutamine, chlorophyll, granular kelp, pantothenic acid, pangamic acid, octacosanol, EPA, amino acids and digestive enzymes. Raw glandulars in tablet form have been of great help to many people. If any gland in your body is not functioning at top speed, you might profit by taking adrenals, thymus, thyroid, ovaries, pituitary or several others, singly or combined. They are available at health food stores.

3

NO MORE JUNK FOOD

LET'S SWITCH

If you're sick of being sick and tired of being tired, and if you want to prevent disease, especially cancer and other chronic diseases, just *Switchover* with this cookbook to natural foods with all their superior flavor and food value. Even if you've never realized the importance of good nutrition for your health, you will probably feel better on this program after only a few days. Most people do. Hundreds of letters in my files attest to more energy, fewer weight problems in people who were over- or underweight and fewer illnesses, even the big one—cancer.

If you have cancer now, one of the main differences between your old food program and your new one based on this book is that cancer patients don't eat animal protein for a while, except a little yogurt. Otherwise, to *prevent* cancer, we eat a natural food diet with moderate amounts of animal protein, small amounts of excellent fat and large amounts of plant protein and complex carbohydrates. All of these foods contain vitamins and minerals in maximum amounts. This diet helps keep our immune system strong enough to destroy precancerous cells before they can grow into tumors.

It's a wonderful new life—you'll be peppy, slim and healthy. But you may need some suggestions about how to switch.

They're in this book.

This book incorporates the easiest ways to change from junk food to good food. Every suggestion for change includes the reason for the change. Every recipe is easy to make, and it tastes good. Every recipe is quick, easy, delicious and nutritious. All recipes are designed to promote optimal health.

So let's prepare natural food from scratch; let's change from eating junk to eating food. Most of all, let's do it easily and enjoy it.

Just because we cook from scratch doesn't mean we spend a lot of time in the kitchen. We learn tricks to get us out quickly, in less time than before, but the food we eat will taste better and cost less, and every bite will build health.

THE LOWER COST OF NATURAL FOODS

Let's get one question out of the way in a hurry—how does a natural food diet compare in price with the usual American diet from the supermarket? Are we going to be spending a lot more money?

No. The money you save by not eating convenience foods may surprise you. One of my counselees said she had saved $100 the first month on this program. Natural foods are much cheaper than convenience foods. Our main items of food are fish, poultry, eggs, dairy products, whole grains, legumes (beans, peas and peanuts), vegetables, whole fruits, nuts and seeds.

We prepare these foods quickly from scratch. Rather than having someone mix our flour and shortening to make biscuit mix and charge us a high price for it, we mix it ourselves (in seconds, if we have a food processor). We avoid the refined grains, the chemical preservatives and the high prices; and we get whole grains, no preservatives to damage our livers and a much lower price.

The most valuable gain is health. We can't put a price on health. A good diet will keep your child from having an infection which can turn into pneumonia, with possible weakness for life. Can you say, "Wholewheat flour costs more than white flour; I can't afford it"?

HOW MUCH SHOULD WE EAT?

On this program we don't worry about calories or grams because we're all different in size, in how fast we burn food and in how active we are. Let's just not overload our digestive systems. If we aren't hungry enough to enjoy our mext meal or snack, we've eaten too much the time before. You'll soon realize what's right for you. Your brain will help, because it will tell you you've had enough to eat and you won't even want to eat more than your body needs.

If you've ever fought the battle of the bulge, it may be that the section of your brain called the hypothalamus isn't working well because it isn't getting the nutrients it needs to make it healthy. The hypothalamus determines our appestat. Researchers have cut one side of the hypothalamus of rats, which then starved to death with food in front of them. When the other side of the hypothalamus was cut, rats gorged on food until they ate themselves to death.

People who eat junk food or who are overweight may have a damaged hypothalamus which will not be able to set their appestat so they will eat the right amount of food. How can we repair our hypothalamus? By eating excellent food that will repair its tissues.

Also, the hypothalamus obviously sets the *kind* of food we eat. I know people who can eat sweets all the time. Their hypothalamus must not be working well. I also know people who eat small amounts of healthful sweets and are satisfied. If they haven't had a fresh raw salad for a day, they crave one. They may crave a whole grain muffin, a cup of cool refreshing yogurt, or a bowl of flavorful fish chowder. Thus nature will take care of our food requirements if we cooperate and eat to keep our brain cells healthy (Williams, 1971).

Most people lose weight gradually on this diet. A man called me on the phone one day and said, "I've been on your diet six weeks and have lost ten pounds." I said, "I hope you wanted to." "Yes," he said, "I needed to lose, but I don't want to lose ten pounds every six weeks." But everyone gets to a plateau that's right for them.

If you need to gain when you start this diet, eat a little more fat (butter, cream, eggs, nuts and seeds) and go up on carbohydrates, especially potatoes, sweet potatoes and legumes.

TYPES OF NATURAL FOODS

What is the big difference between our natural food diet and the average American diet?

On a natural food diet, we don't eat a lot of red meat (muscle meat—steaks, roasts, chops and hamburger). We use red meat as a condiment—a little goes a long way. Most nutritionists suggest no more than four ounces of red meat four times a week, but we don't have to eat that much. Less is better, and most of us can get along without any. But we need excellent protein from animal and vegetable sources.

We should buy our chickens at health food stores, because commercial chickens are fed many additives, especially growth hormone, pesticides that get in their feed and antibiotics to keep down infections.

We may eat one or two eggs a day and cook with extra eggs (from the health food store). The cholesterol myth has been exploded. The body manufactures cholesterol, and the more we eat, the less we have to manufacture. If we get all the nutrients we need, our cholesterol will be manufactured in the amounts we need and no more.

Dairy proteins—whole milk, yogurt and kefir (soured milks), and cheeses (natural and light colored to avoid orange chemical dyes) —are good in moderate amounts.

We eat a lot of plant proteins, whole grains, nuts and seeds—combined with legumes (beans, peas and peanuts).

We eat vegetables both cooked and raw, and whole, fresh, raw, ripe fruit.

For the oil and fat we need, we nibble nuts and seeds with each of our six small meals. Nuts and seeds are important sources of linoleic acid, the one essential fatty acid the body can't manufacture. "Nibbles" of nuts and seeds are one to two teaspoons of sesame, sunflower or pumpkin seeds, two walnut halves, four pecan halves, six almonds or twelve peanuts. If we eat one of these small portions six times a day, we won't gain weight, and we will get the linoleic acid that's essential to our health. We don't eat oil from a bottle; the chemical structure of the oil has been changed by the processing, and it no longer fits the chemistry of our cells. Our livers can detoxify poisons if there aren't too many of them, so use little or no oil-based dressings. Use them only when you're at a friend's house or a restaurant. At home, use the dressings recommended in this book.

We eat wholegrain foods. We can eat a biscuit, muffin, cracker or a small piece of bread we've made ourselves from whole grains.

It isn't much fun to eat if we just open cans, and it isn't possible to cook fancy meals all the time; we'd wear ourselves out. But when we prepare natural foods simply and healthfully, food preparation becomes a pleasure.

A man called me one day to say he had got hold of one of my books on diet. He said, "My wife and I are having fun planning our meals. In fact, it's the most fun I've had. I used to think photography and loading my own ammunition were the most fun, but now I like working out this diet." I know what photography is, but I didn't know what he meant about the ammunition. He said, "I'm a skeet shooter, and I used to like loading my own ammunition more than anything; but now we are having so much fun with this way of eating, I just wanted to call and tell you."

Note that he said "fun"—perhaps the family that cooks together is happy together.

FOOD FOR OUR BRAINS

Preparing food for our families *is* fun and rewarding, especially when we realize its importance for the health of our brains. Good food determines our emotions and our personalities. If you have anyone with an obnoxious personality or with emotional problems, he or she will change for the better on a good diet.

And this diet is the best "treatment" in the world for divorce-minded couples! They may not realize that a deficiency of nutrients can cause confusion, fatigue, irritability, and other mental problems from poor concentration to stuporous depression.

And think of the children who suffer from these very problems. They aren't happy and don't know why—they don't want to be the way they are. They deserve good food to make their brain cells healthy so their minds will be happy. Don't you owe this chance for peace and contentment to your own family?

PRACTICAL MENUS

By planning ahead at odd times, we prepare food for the next day or the next meal. We give the kids special jobs—growing sprouts, making crackers, washing vegetables; and if the wife works, the husband helps cook. Some husbands I know make the bread once a month or so and keep the freezer full of muffins, bread, biscuits and crackers. If this is a family project, everybody will be interested, and everybody will feel good.

We always prepare vegetables for only one meal at a time, but we cook grains and legumes ahead, since it's just as easy to cook large amounts as small. We freeze meal-size portions and are ready for many quick, delicious, healthful meals.

This plan can be adjusted for any size family. You're used to the amounts of staples, fruits and vegetables your family eats in a week, so buy the usual amounts.

KITCHEN PLANNING

To cook easily, we may need to rearrange a few things. We can start with the freezer. My favorite "file drawers" for the freezer are bicycle baskets. They are cheaper than freezer baskets, and they work just as well. You may want to label the baskets "raw grains," "cooked grains," "legumes," "raw fish," "cooked proteins" (such as millet burgers, meat loaf, grain loaf, etc.). Also "pureed fruits and fruit juices" for making jellies.

Use a basket for all your flours and other dry ingredients for baking. They'll be handy—

one quick trip from freezer to counter and all dry ingredients are ready. The liquid ingredients—butter, eggs and milk—require another quick trip from fridge to counter.

Find a spot for nuts and seeds. They stay in the shelves on the door of the fridge at my house. But they don't stay there very long because everyone helps himself to small amounts several times a day.

FOOD SUPPLEMENTS

In addition to as good food as we can get, most of us need food supplements in order to be healthy. For a food supplement program for adults and children, those who may or may not have serious health problems now and definitely want to avoid problems in the future, see Lesson 1 in my book, *A Home Study Course in the New Nutrition.*

Others of the twelve lessons describe specific supplements for serious health problems such as allergies, heart disease, high and low blood sugar, aging, arthritis, children's problems, mental abnormalities, depression and weight control. This course is available from the Nutrition Education Association, Inc., P. O. Box 20301, Houston, Texas 77225, phone 713/665-2946.

GETTING READY

One of the most important things I can say about food is "Don't eat too much at one time." You can digest and assimilate your food well, and you'll have an appetite for the next meal or mid-meal if you eat small amounts. Eat slowly and chew each bite many times. Sometimes this alone will get you over such problems as gas and indigestion and off to a good start on your new way of life.

This food plan may look like more cooking than you've been doing, and you're afraid you'll be in the kitchen all day when you see the diet written out like this. You won't be. Mid-meals are pick-up meals, and everybody picks up his own. Business people and students will take nibble food with them for snacks. Once in a while, I hear that school teachers and administrators won't let children eat between meals.

Tell them that nutritious snacks are required for their health, on orders from their nutritionist. If all teachers and students ate healthful snacks, everyone would soon realize that people do not get tired or irritable or become fuzzy thinkers if they nibble good food throughout the day. Their blood sugar will be level— not too high or too low; they will be peppy and cooperative.

SHOPPING LIST

Here's a shopping list for the first two weeks, to get you started.

FROM HEALTH FOOD STORE

honey	dark brown sugar
sea salt	vegetable salt
eggs	wholewheat flour
millet	wheat flakes
wheat germ	stone ground cornmeal
unrefined bran	buckwheat
oatmeal	seven-grain cereal
soy powder	four-grain cereal
baking powder	non-instant powdered
carob powder	milk
baker's yeast	lecithin granules
peanut butter	plain yogurt (or
soy flakes	culture to make
coconut	your own)
carob chips	organically grown
seeds to sprout (alfalfa	carrots
and mung bean)	seeds to eat (sunflower,
raisins, other dried	sesame and
fruit	pumpkin)
chicken	turkey
apple cider vinegar	

Buy fresh vegetables and fruits, natural cheese, dried beans and peas, and dairy products from health food stores if they have them— otherwise from the supermarket. Buy all eggs and chickens, whole grains and carrots from health food stores. (Most of these stores sell organically grown, delicious carrots.) Most people don't realize that health food stores sell chickens, but they do, and they taste so much better than the ordinary chickens, you'll never go back to the old kind. We don't buy processed foods even from health food stores. We prepare everything from scratch.

FROM SUPERMARKET

spices
popcorn
tuna fish
salmon
whole milk
sardines
sweet potatoes
white potatoes
dried beans and peas
 of your choice
fish
lean meat

calves' liver
cheese (natural, light
 colored)
cottage cheese
fresh fruit
fresh vegetables
nuts in shell (or
 shelled), not in cans
 or jars; not salted;
 as many different
 kinds as possible

LIQUIDS TO DRINK

In the following menus, to remind you about drinking water thirty minutes before meals, we include it in the first day's meal plans. After that, you'll know to drink it, and we won't list it every day.

People sometimes ask me how much water to drink. We need different amounts because we're different sizes, and we have different life styles. Some of us perspire more than others, so some need to drink more than others. Your body will tell you if you're drinking enough liquids: you should have soft, well-formed bowel movements, two or three a day. You should have a good flow of urine. You shouldn't drink so much water that you can't eat at meal and mid-meal times. If you wish, drink milk, yogurt, kefir or soup in small amounts with meals.

4

MENUS FOR TWO WEEKS

Abbreviations: t-teaspoon, T-tablespoon, c-cup

In the two weeks of menus we have for you, there are several choices for most meals, so you can please your own taste buds. There are quickie recipes so you won't be in the kitchen all the time.

After you've been into the new way of life for a while, you'll be adventuresome and will try different recipes and menus. The entire program may be *different* from the usual, but it is *not difficult.*

Let's start our two-week sample program on Monday. That will give us the weekend to shop and to prepare a few dishes ahead so we can get into the whole program on a regular work-school day.

After you get the shopping done, make some dishes for the fridge or freezer on Saturday and Sunday. If you have a large enough freezer, prepare large amounts of breads, grains and beans. Otherwise, prepare small amounts for storage in the fridge. Bread is important, so we'll start with easy, delicious muffins. We'll call these dishes "Prepare Ahead."

"Prepare Ahead" on Saturday and Sunday.

1. Favorite muffins p. 77
2. Jump-on crackers p. 79
3. Corn Dodgers, p. 79
4. Pancakes p. 80
5. One-hour, no-hands bread p. 75

These five recipes should be easy to mix up in about an hour. It takes extra time to finish cooking them.

Cook and freeze or refrigerate:
No-Meat Loaf p. 62
Probly-the-Best Brownies, p. 119

Freeze:
Sliced bananas for smoothies p. 101

DAY 1—MONDAY

Each item of food on this chart is marked either "Now," "Ahead" or "Bought."

n) now
a) ahead
b) bought

"Now" means prepare now (at meal time). "Ahead" means the item was prepared ahead and is in the freezer or fridge ready to be warmed up or served. "Bought" means that the food was bought as it will be served. This should help you keep track of the foods you will be preparing, and it will be easy to know how much preparation time will be needed.

The heading marked "a" is a signal to the cook that food is already prepared and can be served immediately or steamed quickly. The next time Junior has a Little League game and time is short, get out the frozen Hamburger Pizza that was first served on Day 2, and you'll realize how quick and easy this meal planning is. You'll eat well, and you'll get to the game on time.

The idea is, every time we prepare a main dish, if we prepare enough for two, four or six meals, we'll realize that food in the freezer is like money in the bank. We'll have our convenience foods, but they will build health with every bite.

30 MINUTES BEFORE BREAKFAST:

6 to 12 ounces water (depending on individual need) at room temperature

BREAKFAST:
n) 1 or 2 poached or soft boiled eggs, hardboiled if not overcooked, or scrambled in butter in a moderate (not hot) skillet
a) Favorite muffins

30 MINUTES BEFORE SNACK:
6 to 12 ounces water

MID-MORNING SNACK:
b) ½ to 1 inch cube of light colored, natural cheese, ¼ to ½ apple

30 MINUTES BEFORE LUNCH:
6 to 12 ounces water

LUNCH:
b) peanut butter sandwich (p. 133)
a) on whole wheat bread (p. 74)
n) tossed vegetable salad (p. 94)

30 MINUTES BEFORE SNACK:
6 to 12 ounces water

MID-AFTERNOON SNACK:
b) mixed nuts
b) ¼ to 1 orange

30 MINUTES BEFORE SUPPER:
6 to 12 ounces water

SUPPER:
a) No-Meat Loaf (p. 62)
n) with tomato sauce (p. 28)
n) or cheese sauce (p. 29)
n) Steamed carrots (p. 90)
n) with butter
b) or with chopped mixed nuts

30 MINUTES BEFORE SNACK:
6 to 12 ounces water

EVENING SNACK:
n) banana smoothie, bananas frozen ahead (p. 101)

"Prepare Ahead" on Monday

While the children (or husband) are loading the dishwasher, make hamburger pizza (p. 43) and salad dressing (pp. 96–98). Cook beans and grains so you will be ready to mix Bean and Grain Burgers tomorrow (p. 65).

You get the idea about drinking water before meals. You'll soon get the habit, and you won't have to be reminded to drink. We won't list the water before meals after this, but don't forget to drink it.

One of my counselees who had a long-standing problem—halitosis—said that after she changed her diet and drank water all day like this, she got completely over her bad breath. Another said she was no longer constipated when she drank her water before meals. Many people have told me that there is "immediate relief" from gas and bloating when they don't drink liquids with meals. This is because the hydrochloric acid in the stomach doesn't get so diluted. Good digestion of protein calls for strong stomach acid.

DAY 2—TUESDAY

BREAKFAST:
a) Wholegrain pancake (p. 81)
b) pile on top: cottage cheese, fresh fruit, yogurt and a sprinkle of nuts

SNACK:
a) Favorite muffin (p. 77)
b) with peanut butter
b) fresh orange sections

LUNCH:
b) hard cheese
a) on Corn Dodger (p. 79)
n) vegetable salad (p. 94)
a) salad dressing (p. 96)

SNACK:
a) Jump-on cracker (p. 79)
b) half (or less) banana

SUPPER:
a) Hamburger pizza—eat half, freeze half (p. 43)
n) steamed vegetables; cabbage (p. 88), or broccoli (greens), p. 89)

SNACK:
a) brownie (p. 119)
b) apple or peach

"Prepare Ahead" on Tuesday

Mix Bean or Grain Burgers (p. 65). Leave in fridge to bake for Wednesday supper. Cook turkey thighs overnight in slow cooker or steam in cooker-steamer when you get home from work. Before bed, remove turkey from bones, store in fridge.

Cook overnight in thermos: breakfast grains (p. 81). Prepare tuna fish sandwiches. Freeze for those who carry lunch.

DAY 3—WEDNESDAY

BREAKFAST:
n) 1 or 2 eggs
a) whole grains cooked in thermos (p. 81)

SNACK:
a) bread or cracker
b) with peanuts
b) ¼ to 1 apple

LUNCH:
n) Tuna fish sandwich (filling prepared ahead)
a) on whole wheat toast or bread
b) carrot and celery sticks with cashews

SNACK:
b) 1 inch cube of hard cheese
b) ¼ to 1 orange

SUPPER:
a) Cook Bean or Grain Burgers (p. 65) (eat half and freeze half)
b) Melt grated cheese over the burgers
n) Steamed greens (p. 89)

SNACK:
n) Banana smoothie (bananas frozen ahead) (p. 101)
b) six almonds

"Prepare Ahead" on Wednesday

Mix Fowl Is Fair recipe (p. 47) ready for steaming for Thursday supper. Cook brown rice (it takes one hour). Freeze or refrigerate: corn muffins (p. 78), angel food cake (p. 115).

DAY 4—THURSDAY

BREAKFAST:
n) Quickie Egg Drink (p. 107)
a) Favorite muffin (p. 77)

SNACK:
b) small cube of hard cheese
b) prunes or other fruit

LUNCH:
n) Talk-show liver (p. 45)
n) Vegetable salad (p. 94)

SNACK:
a) High-protein angel food cake (p. 115)
b) 3 to 6 almonds
b) ¼ to 1 apple

SUPPER:
a) Fowl Is Fair turkey
a) served on brown rice (eat half, freeze half)
n) Steamed squash—summer (p. 89), winter (p. 91)

SNACK:
b) yogurt (p. 51)
n) or carob nut milk (p. 107)
b) half banana

"Prepare Ahead" on Thursday

Cook and freeze in serving portions or refrigerate: Millet (p. 62), red beans (p. 65), trail mix (p. 126). Freeze fruit for smoothies.

DAY 5—FRIDAY

BREAKFAST:
a) Trail mix (p. 126)
b) with milk or yogurt (p. 51)
n) Scrambled egg

SNACK:
b) Cube of cheese
b) Fresh fruit

LUNCH:
a) Hamburger pizza (p. 43)
n) green vegetable salad (p. 94)

SNACK:
a) Brownie
b) Fresh fruit

SUPPER:
n) Millet frizzled in butter, topped with sesame seeds, millet already prepared (p. 62)
n) Red bean salad (p. 95), beans already cooked

SNACK:
n) Fruit smoothie, fruit already frozen (p. 101)
a) Angel food cake (p. 115)

"Prepare Ahead" on Friday

Cook and freeze or refrigerate: Carob Chews (p. 119) and granola (p. 83).

DAY 6—SATURDAY

BREAKFAST:
a) Home-made granola (p. 83)
b) Milk or yogurt (p. 51)

SNACK:
b) Cottage cheese
b) Fresh fruit

LUNCH:
a) No-Meat Loaf (p. 62)
n) Slaw with toasted cashews (p. 95)

SNACK:
a) Carob chews (p. 119)
b) Fresh fruit

SUPPER:
n) Cheese fondue (p. 49)
n) Steamed broccoli or other vegetable
n) with nut milk sauce (p. 28)

SNACK:
b) Yogurt (p. 51)
n) or carob nut milk (p. 107)
b) Fresh fruit

"Prepare Ahead"

Take Saturday evening off!

DAY 7—SUNDAY

BREAKFAST:
n) Quickie Egg Drink (p. 107)
a) Favorite muffins (p. 77)

SNACK:
b) Cube of natural cheese
b) Fresh fruit

LUNCH:
a) Grain and Bean Burgers (p. 65)
b) Raw vegetables and nuts

SNACK:
b) Milk or yogurt (p. 51)
b) Fresh fruit

SUPPER:
n) Tuna Chowder (p. 46)
   Eat half and freeze half.
n) Steamed cabbage (p. 88)
b) with sunflower seeds
a) Bread or muffins

SNACK:
n) Frozen fruit smoothie (p. 101)
   Fruit frozen ahead
a) Brownie (p. 119)

"Prepare Ahead" on Sunday

Hard boil eggs. Mix and cook till nearly done: Hamburgers for Health (p. 42). Cook overnight in thermos: whole grain cereal (p. 81). Toast peanuts about 20 minutes at 300 F.

DAY 8—MONDAY

BREAKFAST:
a) Cereal cooked in thermos (p. 81)
b) Milk or yogurt (p. 51)

SNACK:
a) Corn Dodger (p. 79)
b) with peanut butter
b) Fresh fruit

LUNCH:
n) Vegetable salad
with hard-boiled egg (p. 94)
a) Favorite muffin (p. 77)

SNACK:
b) Hard cheese,
natural and light colored
b) Fresh fruit

SUPPER:
a) Hamburgers for Health (p. 42)
a) with tomato sauce (p. 28)
n) Steamed carrots with walnuts (p. 90)

SNACK:
n) Popcorn
a) and toasted peanuts
b) Fresh fruit

"Prepare Ahead" on Monday

Cook and freeze or refrigerate: Easy-iced cake (p. 119), cook and refrigerate: brown rice (p. 61).

DAY 9—TUESDAY

BREAKFAST:
n) 1 or 2 eggs
a) Pancake with butter (p. 80)

SNACK:
b) Milk or yogurt (p. 51)
b) Fresh fruit

LUNCH:
n) Talk-show liver (p. 45)
b) Carrot and celery sticks
a) with toasted peanuts

SNACKS:
a) Trail mix (p. 126)
b) Fresh fruit

SUPPER:
a) Fowl Is Fair (p. 47)
a) on brown rice (p. 61)
n) Steamed vegetable combination (p. 91)

SNACK:
a) Easy-iced cake (p. 119)
b) Fresh fruit

"Prepare Ahead" on Tuesday

Prepare sandwich spread of your choice (p. 133). Make nut milk sauce (p. 28).

DAY 10—WEDNESDAY

BREAKFAST:
n) Quickie Egg Drink (p. 107)
b) or yogurt (p. 51)
a) Favorite or corn muffin (pp. 77–78)

SNACK:
b) Mixed nuts and seeds
b) Fresh fruit

LUNCH:
n) Sandwich
(filling prepared ahead p. 133)
a) on whole grain bread (pp. 74–76)
n) Salad of celery and tomatoes or avocados

SNACK:
b) Milk
a) and cracker (pp. 78–79)
b) with peanut butter
b) Fresh fruit

SUPPER:
n) Oven-fried fish (p. 45)
n) Steamed greens or other vegetables (p. 89)

SNACK:
a) Brownie (p. 119)
b) Fresh fruit

"Prepare Ahead" on Wednesday

Make and freeze or refrigerate: crepes (p. 64). Prepare and refrigerate crepe filling (p. 64). Cook in thermos: whole grain cereal (p. 81). Prepare and refrigerate: Linda's dressing (p. 97).

DAY 11—THURSDAY

BREAKFAST:
a) Cereal cooked in thermos (p. 81)
n) One or two eggs

SNACK:
a) Carob chews (p. 119)
b) Fresh fruit

LUNCH:
a) Sandwich on whole wheat bread or muffin
a) Filling prepared ahead (p. 133)
n) Tossed vegetable salad (p. 94)
a) Linda's dressing (p. 97)

SNACK:
b) Milk or yogurt (p. 51)
b) Fresh fruit

SUPPER:
a) Wholegrain crepes
a) with cottage cheese or vegetable
    filling (p. 64)
a) and nut milk sauce (p. 28)
n) Steamed broccoli or other vegetable (p. 89)

SNACK:
a) Easy-iced cake (p. 118)
b) Fresh fruit

"Prepare Ahead" on Thursday

   Bake and replace in freezer any bread, crackers, biscuits or muffins in short supply.

DAY 12—FRIDAY

BREAKFAST:
a) Trail mix (p. 126)
b) with yogurt (p. 51) or whole milk
b) Cottage cheese

SNACK:
b) Mixed nuts
b) Fresh fruit

LUNCH:
a) Hamburgers for Health (p. 42)
n) Raw vegetables
a) with Vegetable Dressing (p. 97)

SNACK:
b) Peanut butter
a) and crackers (pp. 78–79)
b) Fresh fruit

SUPPER:
n) Tuna Chowder (p. 46)
n) Steamed vegetables with herbs (p. 89)

SNACK:
a) Carob Chews (p. 119)
    or Brownie (p. 119)
b) Fresh fruit

"Prepare Ahead" on Friday

   Skin chicken for Your Own Oven-Fried Chicken (p. 47). Prepare nut sauce (p. 28). Bake sweet potatoes.

DAY 13—SATURDAY

BREAKFAST:
a) Easy Wheat Pancakes (p. 81)
n) 1 or 2 eggs

SNACK:
b) Cottage cheese
b) Fresh fruit

LUNCH:
n) Sandwich (p. 133)
n) Combination vegetable salad (p. 94)
a) with dressing (pp. 96–98)

SNACK:
b) Mixed nuts
b) Fresh fruit

SUPPER:
n) Millet Soufflé (p. 61), millet prepared ahead
n) Steamed vegetables (p. 89)
a) with nut sauce (p. 28)

SNACK:
n) Frozen fruit smoothie (p. 101), fruit frozen
    ahead

"Prepare Ahead" on Saturday

   Take Saturday evening off!

DAY 14—SUNDAY

BREAKFAST:
n) One or two eggs
a) Wholegrain toast or muffin

SNACK:
b) Hard cheese
b) Fresh fruit

LUNCH:
n) Frizzled Fish (p. 46)
n) Sweet potatoes, mashed
n) Steamed cauliflower
n) with cream sauce (p. 27)
b) or herbs and seeds (p. 30)

SNACK:
a) Carob Chews (pp. 119)
b) Fresh fruit

SUPPER:
n) Your Own Oven-Fried Chicken (p. 47)
n) Combination salad (p. 91)

SNACK:
a) Trail mix (p. 126)
b) Fresh fruit

"Prepare Ahead" on Sunday

Take Sunday off!

SUMMING UP

Now we've been through fourteen days of our new way of life, and we should be used to the new foods. From now on, we can use the recipes in this book or in many other good cookbooks and prepare food ahead at the times best for us. Therefore, we'll never have to open cans in an emergency. Our expert planning has resulted in emergency food always being available.

One more idea: Keep on hand some favorite high protein staple foods, prepared and ready to eat. For example, homemade pimento cheese, egg salad (this can help out any meal, especially if you don't have eggs for breakfast), peanut butter, small cans of sardines or kippered snacks. (Canned fish is acceptable.) These protein foods may make a meal in an emergency or add protein to any meal.

You may be wondering what you'll do when you eat out or entertain friends in your home or go to their homes for a meal. There's a way to handle all that—see Eating Out, p. 131, and Entertaining Friends, p. 132. Your friends may not be used to eating good bread, so when you have guests in your home, make rolls, muffins, biscuits or bread from whole grains. You'll get tons of compliments.

Let's enjoy the foods, even if they're new to us. You'll have the pleasure of eating natural foods with their own natural flavors.

5

MAIN DISH SAUCES

Sauces should start the major recipe section of this book, because they can be used on dishes made with animal proteins, plant proteins, and on vegetables, if you wish. Dessert sauces are in the dessert section. If you've never eaten nut sauces, here's a whole new idea opening up for you.

You'll probably eat more of your steamed vegetables with just a little butter to bring out the flavor. One of my counselees was a gourmet cook and liked fancy sauces on everything. About two weeks after seeing me, he called and said he hadn't made a sauce for any vegetable since. He added, "I don't mask the delicate flavors of the vegetables with sauce. They don't need it." You may occasionally need a gourmet sauce on protein dishes. Most of these sauces are happy additions to meats, fish, grains, and legumes.

High protein sauces are made with milk, yogurt, buttermilk, hard-boiled eggs, cheese, nuts and/or seeds. While vegetables are still in the steamer, pour on a little buttermilk or yogurt. Transfer to serving dish and grate cheese on top. Add chopped hard-boiled egg, and sprinkle on some seeds or nuts. Broccoli, peas and cauliflower are especially good with almonds, walnuts and cashews.

Try any of the recipes for salad dressings as sauces on steamed vegetables or on grain and bean loaves and patties.

CREAM SAUCE

To make cream sauce, use the following proportions:

	whole wheat flour	non-instant powdered milk	whole milk
Thin:	1 T	2 T	1 cup
Medium:	2 T	2 T	1 cup
Thick:	3 T	2 T	1 cup

Blend in blender in this order: milk, powdered milk, flour. Heat, stirring constantly until thick. Add 1 T butter and ¼ t or more (to taste) of vegetable or sea salt.
Yield: 1½ cups
Variations: Use part milk and part vegetable stock.

Or: Use arrowroot or cornstarch instead of the wholewheat flour. These thickeners make a smooth, light sauce.

Or: Use buttermilk or yogurt instead of milk. Don't cook soured milks. Blend 1 T butter with 1 T flour in a moderate skillet. Add 1 c buttermilk; warm it only.

Or: Season sauce with frizzled mushrooms, herbs and spices (coriander, mustard powder or curry).

Or: Season with grated onion, 2 T Lemon juice, and 4 T grated Parmesan cheese. Pour a small amount of sauce over two beaten eggs in a small bowl, stir, and return to heat for a few minutes. Excellent on green vegetables.

BEAN GRAVY

Juice from cooked dried beans is rich and tasty and can be eaten with baked potatoes or other vegetables. Thicken it by blending some of the whole beans with the juice and seasoning it with a pinch of dried ginger, a little garlic and toasted sesame seeds.

LEMONY BUTTER SAUCE

Combine in a blender:
    Juice of 1 lemon
    grated peel of half the lemon
    ½ c melted butter
Serve on vegetables.
Yield: ⅝ cup

BETTER THAN SOUR CREAM

Mix well in blender and chill:
    ½ c milk
    1 c thick yogurt
    ½ c cottage cheese
    2 T lemon juice
Yield: 2 cups

SOUR CREAM WITH GELATIN

Blend:
    1 c hot water from faucet
    1 T gelatin
Add:
    3 egg yolks
    ½ c whole milk
    1 T vinegar
    1 t each honey and vegetable salt
Use over lettuce or baked potato.
Yield: 1½ cups
Variation: omit vinegar, use only a pinch of salt.

NUT MILK

Nut milks make super sauces for millet or bean burgers, wheat loaves or steamed vegetables.

In blender, grind to a powder:
    ½ c any nuts
If you use peanuts, toast them first. Other nuts and seeds can be used raw. Gradually add 1 c water or more—to the consistency you like. Pour over food in serving dish. If you have leftover sauces, pour them in the soup jar in the freezer.
Yield: 1½ cups

CREAM OF SESAME SAUCE

Mix together then pour into blender:
    ½ c tahini (sesame butter)
    1 c cold water
Add and blend until smooth:
    Tamari soy sauce to taste
    juice of ½ lemon
    ½ T fresh chopped parsley
    ½ clove garlic minced
    1 T honey
Store in airtight bottle in fridge. Serve on fish, vegetables, potatoes.
Yield: 1½ cups

TOMATO SAUCE

Easy to make, and it contains very little sugar.

Combine in a processor, steel blade:
    12 large home-frozen or fresh ripe tomatoes, peeled (p. 86)
    1 onion, quartered
    2 T chopped fresh basil or ½ t powdered basil
    2 green peppers, seeded
    2 to 3 sprigs parsley
    6 ribs celery in chunks
    2 cloves garlic
Process till pureed. In large cooker, bring to a boil, simmer uncovered 45 minutes. Store overnight in fridge so the flavors can blend. Freeze in small containers if you wish.
Yield: 8 cups.

QUICK TOMATO SAUCE

In blender:
    1½ cups home-frozen or fresh tomatoes, peeled (p. 86)
    ½ t salt
    ⅛ t cumin powder
    ⅛ t pepper
    ½ c apple cider vinegar
    ½ t oregano
    ⅛ t nutmeg
    1 t salad mustard

Blend and chill. Add water to desired consistency.
Yield: 2 cups

NUTTY PIMENTO CHEESE SAUCE WITHOUT THE CHEESE

Blend all ingredients in blender:
 1 c water
 ¾ c cashew nuts or sunflower seeds
 2 T sesame seeds
 1¼ t salt
 3 T brewer's yeast flakes
 1 t onion powder
 ⅛ t garlic powder
 ⅛ dill seed
 ½ c pimentos
 ¼ c lemon juice (or to taste)
Yield: 2¾ cups
To make into brick for sliced "cheese" sandwiches, mix well and boil until flakes are dissolved:
 6 T agar flakes or 2 T agar powder
 1 ½ c water
Add to ingredients in blender; mix and blend till creamy. Pour into mold and chill.

CHEESE SAUCE

Blend in blender, then pour into small saucepan, heat and stir till thick:
 1 c milk
 2 T flour
Add and stir over low heat till cheese is melted:
 ¾ c grated light colored cheddar cheese
 ½ t salt
 1 t paprika
 ½ t dry mustard
 2 T butter
Yield: 2 cups

GARBANZO BEAN SAUCE

Mix in saucepan over medium heat. Stir till warm and butter is melted:
 1 c cooked garbanzo beans, mashed
 1 t vegetable broth powder
 1 T lemon juice
 1 T butter
 salt and pepper to taste
Yield: 1⅛ cups

MOSTLY FRUIT RELISH

Relish made with fresh and dried fruits and vegetables is a super topping for pancakes, waffles and biscuits. It fills cream puff shells well when mixed with cottage cheese and/or yogurt. It goes so well with grain and bean patties and tofu patties that you might save it for that. But don't save it; eat it.

Combine in a large kettle:
 3 c organically grown dried peaches, raisins, apricots (or other fruits of your choice)
 two large grated carrots (organically grown, from your health food store)
 two or three peeled, grated apples.
Simmer until the carrots and apples are almost mush. This keeps well in the freezer.

CRANBERRY SAUCE PLUS

Simmer for 15 minutes in a large saucepan:
 1 pound washed cranberries
 1½ c water
 ¾ c dark brown sugar (recipe p. 109)
 1 orange cut into sections (remove seeds and the orange rind—leave some of the white rind)
 1 c raisins
 ½ c chopped celery
 ½ c chopped walnuts or pecans
 ½ t ground ginger (optional)
Pour into glass jars, cool, and refrigerate or freeze. Serve with turkey or almost any other meat or plant protein loaf or patties.
Yield: 6 cups.

QUICK AND EASY SAUCE THICKENER

Here's another quick trick.

Place in a bowl until butter is soft:
 ½ c butter
 ½ c whole wheat flour or cornstarch
Mix well and drop by tablespoons on foil covered tray (dull side of foil next to food). When frozen, place in plastic bags. Use to thicken sauces and gravies. The cornstarch thickener is nice in Chinese vegetable dishes.
Yield: 8 drops, 2 T each

DEVILED SAUCE

Combine and mix well:
  ⅓ c apple cider vinegar
  ⅓ c melted butter
  1 t Worcestershire sauce
  ½ t salt
  ½ t paprika
  ½ t dry mustard
Serve on vegetables.
Yield: ¾ cup

BUTTERMILK MUSTARD SAUCE

Mix together in blender:
  1 c buttermilk
  2 T salad mustard (or to taste)
  1 peeled apple cut in chunks
Heat (do not boil) and serve on steamed vegetables.
Yield: 1½ cups

VEGGIE TOPPING

Stir and sauté:
  1 c wholegrain bread crumbs (or half wheat germ)
  ⅓ c butter
Add if you wish:
  minced onion
  chopped parsley
  chopped nuts
Yield: 1½ cups

DRAWN BUTTER

Mix well in small skillet:
  4 T melted butter
  1 T lemon juice or Worcestershire sauce
  4 T minced parsley or chive
  Serve on potatoes or other vegetable.
Yield: about ½ cup

BECHAMEL SAUCE

Melt in small pan over medium heat:
  2 T butter
Stir in and blend:
  1½ to 2 T flour

Gradually stir in:
  ½ c hot milk
  ½ c light colored meat or vegetable stock
Cook and stir sauce until it is smooth and boiling. Season it with salt and paprika.
Yield: 1¼ cups

Variation: Add an egg yolk. First, put a little sauce into the yolk, then stir it into the rest of the sauce, then stir until the sauce thickens slightly. Do not boil after adding the yolk.

GARNISHES FOR SAUCE

Choose a peppy "additive" for any sauce. Here are many choices:

  chopped parsley
  capers
  caraway seeds
  slightly steamed chopped celery
  celery seeds
  dill seeds
  sliced stuffed olives
  finely chopped steamed carrots
  chopped chives
  grated lemon rind
  toasted sesame seeds
  curry powder
  garlic
  onions
  chopped hard-cooked eggs
  horseradish
  chopped pickles
  nutmeg
  sherry
  Parmesan cheese
  green pepper
  toasted peanuts
  sunflower seeds or almonds soaked in ice water for 15 minutes

6

ANIMAL PROTEINS

We eat proteins, first, last, and in between. The word "protein" means "of first importance." But to prevent cancer and other diseases, we eat only moderate amounts of red meat—muscle meat (steak, roasts, chops and hamburger) no more than four ounces four times a week, preferably less. When we eat meat moderately, we digest food better, and it helps keep our immune system working well. Undigested proteins are poison in our cells, and they can travel in the blood all over the body, causing disease wherever they land.

We don't eat any animal proteins if we have active cancer. We should choose grains and beans with a little yogurt for our proteins. The plant proteins are discussed at length in Chapter 8, Plant Protein Main Dishes, and in Chapter 9, Bread and Breakfast Grains. Beef is the most tainted meat; commercial chicken is not far behind because of the growth hormone, pesticides and antibiotics in their feed. Buy your chickens at the health food store. They cost more, but they're worth it. Use chicken and red meat as condiments to flavor other foods, as the Chinese and Mexicans do.

Fish is excellent protein; man doesn't usually feed fish hormones or additives to make them fat. If we can buy the fish fresh from the sea, it's good food. Frozen fish is usually acceptable. Don't buy the kind that has been coated with crumbs or flour.

Eggs are also excellent protein, although we've been told for twenty or thirty years not to eat them. It is now known that our bodies manufacture cholesterol because we have to have it. It's part of our brains, sex glands, adrenal glands, and part of every cell in our bodies. If we eat more cholesterol, we make

less; and if we eat less, we make more. One or two eggs a day are suggested, and we can cook with extra eggs.

Dairy products are good sources of protein. Adults should probably drink no more than two glasses of milk a day, one of them yogurt. We eat natural, light-colored cheese, such as Swiss, mozzarella, Monterey Jack. These have no orange dyes.

Some of the best proteins for prevention as well as control of cancer are those from plants, which we'll talk about in the next section.

MUSCLE MEATS

When we shop for meat, we need to know that other parts of the animal have more food value than muscle meats. The best nutrition for our dollar is lamb or beef kidney; it has more protein than any other meat (Walczak, 1977). Utility beef is good; beef heart has more food value than other muscle meats. Strip bacon and filet mignon give the least value for your money. The leanest meat with the highest proportion of polyunsaturated fatty acids is from free-range animals.

GRADES

When we buy meat, we may see grades stamped on it by the U. S. government. The highest grade is U. S. Prime, but it is not often available. U. S. Choice is very acceptable; it is what is found in the meat department of supermarkets. It has fat marbled through, and it tastes good. Commercial grade is usually from older animals. It has a thick fat covering, but it is not very tender.

If the meat isn't graded, it is of high quality if the lean meat is light red, velvety-appearing, and has much fat marbled through it. The bones are pink and white, and the fat is flaky and white. The darker the meat, the older the animal (Walczak, 1977). Most nutritionists say don't eat prime steak; it is marbled with fat which is full of pesticides. Standard is the best grade, because it has very little fat (Nichols, 1972). Lean ham has 25 percent of its calories as protein and 75 percent as fat; lean choice trimmed sirloin is 65 percent protein and 35 percent fat—untrimmed, it is 24 percent protein, 76 percent fat (Ballentine, 1978).

MEATS TO AVOID

Some meats are best not purchased at all. Pork is a questionable buy. The animals are usually injected with a tranquilizer before slaughter, and that gives them their lovely pink color. There is no grading standard; the amount of fat is appalling. Even canned hams may be spoiled. They must be refrigerated, but many supermarkets don't refrigerate them (Goldbeck, 1973). If you do eat pork, cook it well done to avoid trichinosis. Don't eat it often (Walczak, 1977).

Frozen pot pies all contain sugar, poor quality starch, and a lot of salt. They have a lot of highly saturated fat.

Gelatin is not a good protein because it has too much glycine for a good amino acid balance (Davis, 1965). That means that there is so much of one amino acid that the rest are in short supply.

WHAT'S WRONG WITH MEAT?

Much meat used today is spoiled. Many samples have clostridium perfringens—bacteria that are killed by heat but leave toxins in the meat. Frankfurters on sale have been examined, and 40 percent were found to be spoiled by bacteria (Ballentine, 1978).

Parasites can be found in meat not well cooked, especially trichina in pork, which can get into beef sliced with knives used for pork. Pesticides and other pollutants accumulate in animal fat.

Meat, fish and poultry contain two and one-half times more DDT and similar pesticides than dairy products, and thirteen times as much as grains and vegetables. Even if DDT is not being used, it is still present in the atmosphere, and the total use of pesticides has increased.

Reducing the amount of meat we eat will help reduce our intake of pesticides, and increasing the amount of fibrous foods will help pull toxic chemicals out of the body (Ballentine, 1978).

The beef from a grain-fed cow is more tender, more tasteless, and fatter than that from a range-fed cow. Freshly killed meat doesn't have much taste, but the flavor gets better during the next twenty-four hours. The meat is aged for about ten days to allow the enzymes to make it tender. Goat meat is eaten in certain areas, but it is inedible if the animal is more than three months old.

Processed meats are not nearly as wholesome as fresh ones. When meat is salted, as bacon is when it is processed, vitamins B1 and B3 are lost. Each American consumes an average of eighty highly processed hot dogs per year.

PREPARATION

First of all, never soak meat to wash it; just pat with a damp paper towel. One of the most important things about cooking meat is to cook it slowly at low temperatures. We should never eat meat raw or overcooked. Proteins in meats aren't easily digested when overcooked. Overcooked proteins stick together, and that makes them so tough that our digestive enzymes can't break them down to amino acids. Moderate heat is best. As for raw meat, the amount of bacteria present is unknown, but it's always there (Goldbeck, 1973).

Basically, there are two ways to cook meat: with dry or moist heat. Roasting and broiling and their variations are examples of dry heat.

A meat loaf is cooked by dry heat. Commercial grade beef is all right to make it with; beef heart ground and mixed with ground beef is nutritious.

Roasting

Roasting is one of the easiest ways of cooking meat. Just put the roast with the fat side up in a pan in a preheated 250 degree F oven. Don't cover it, and don't add liquid, salt or other seasoning.

Although well-marbled meat is tender, we will be buying meat without much marbling because the fat contains poisons from the air, feed and water that the animal takes in while it is grazing. But we do want the meat to be tender, so we cook it at a lower than usual temperature. At 250 degrees F, a 4-pound roast cooked about four hours will be rare. You will need about five hours for medium, and about six hours for well-done. Roasts that are solid or rolled take longer to cook than those that are flat or otherwise not compact.

A good way to season roast beef is by making gravy and adding your favorite spices and herbs to the gravy. Make the gravy ahead of time if you can, and let the fat rise to the top. Skim it off to avoid eating excess fat.

Broiling

To broil meat, don't preheat the broiler. Keep the heat low. Place the meat four to six inches from the heat with the broiler door open. Broil one side, turn and finish cooking. To pan broil, use a heavy skillet; don't add fat, water or salt. Pour off the fat as it accumulates; use low heat. To sauté, use only enough butter or clarified butter (p. 130) to keep food from sticking. Use flour if you wish. Cook over moderate heat for one to two minutes on each side, then reduce heat to low. If you use an electric range, move the pan to another burner on low and finish cooking.

Braising

Braising and stewing are the basic ways of cooking by moist heat. Braising is cooking by steam. The meat is browned on all sides without grease on low heat in a heavy pan. It can be coated with flour and browned with a small amount of butter in the pan. Then it is placed on a rack, and a small amount of stock or water is added. A little lemon juice or vinegar can be added to the water; it makes the meat more tender. It can be braised in a 200 degree F oven after browning and placing on the rack.

Stewing

Stewing is the other moist-heat way of cooking. It is a variation of braising. The only difference is that water is added, and the meat is cooked in the water, not on a rack. Cuts used are shank, brisket and neck, which can be commercial grade since the meat will be cooked very slowly for a long time. Soups, also, are stews. The muscle meats used for soup have enough flavor to still taste good when some flavor has seeped into the liquid.

Stew meat may be slowly seared with flour or without or not seared at all. Salt is added at the beginning of cooking so the juices will go into the gravy for better flavor. Stew should not be overcooked; the meat should be tender enough to cut with a fork, but it shouldn't fall apart. Beef heart can be stewed or cooked in soup, then cut up and added back to the soup with vegetables (Davis, 1947).

Freezing and Thawing

In preparing frozen meat, don't thaw it completely before cooking it. However, if you need to defrost it for a special recipe, put it in the fridge to thaw. Don't defrost it under running water or at room temperature. These methods destroy nutrients.

Nutrients are found in the drippings when meat thaws. One study showed that the drip from thawed, frozen beef contained 33 percent of the B vitamin pantothenic acid, 15 percent of the niacin, and 8 percent of the folic acid that the meat had before thawing.

ORGAN MEATS

Organ meats are more healthful than muscle meats. Liver contains twenty to fifty times as much B12 as muscle meat; kidneys, ten times as much. We should never refreeze organ meats.

Calves' liver is the best liver. We know that the animal's liver detoxifies poisons it gets in air, food, and water but the liver doesn't store the poisons. Although we can eat calves' liver, we should never eat beef, pork, or chicken livers (Nichols, 1972)—beef liver because the animals have lived long enough to accumulate more toxins than calves; pork liver because pork has trichina; and chicken liver because it may be cancerous.

Veal and lamb kidneys have less "kidney taste." Cook kidneys as little as possible. Cut the white tissue out of the center before washing. Ammonia in the white tissue can penetrate the meat. Bathing the kidneys in a little vinegar will help neutralize the ammonia. Heat speeds up the ammonia production, so cook kidneys at a low temperature a short time (Gerras, 1972).

When cooking brains and sweetbreads, remove the membrane while holding the meat under cool running water. Steam briefly for a salad. If you're sautéing them, don't steam. Broiling saves the delicate flavor of sweetbreads. Brains and sweetbreads usually have to be ordered in advance (Gerras, 1972).

Liver and kidney are lower in fat than muscle meat and equal in protein value. They are higher in iron and vitamins (Seddon and Burrows, 1977).

FISH

Fish is 15 to 20 percent protein of good quality, and its fat is unsaturated. But some fish are as high as 20 percent fat in summer—they feed on plankton near the surface. By the end of winter, they are less than 10 percent fat. White fish such as American sole, which is also called flounder, is low fat. It is better than European flounder. Turbot is another popular white fish.

Shellfish are excellent only when they are fresh and are from unpolluted water. They are high in iron, calcium, B2 and B3. They have only about 3 percent fat and are high in cholesterol. Scallops are about 4 percent carbohydrate; and oysters, 5 percent (Seddon and Burrow, 1977).

PURCHASING

When we buy fish, we get one of the best sources of protein and B vitamins. Choose small ocean fish because they're less polluted, especially halibut (Walczak, 1977).

Fish steaks are cross-section slices of large fish. Fillets are slices off the sides of the fish, cut lengthwise. Both have practically no bone and very little waste.

To judge the freshness of fish, look for eyes that are bright, clear, and bulging; gills that are reddish pink and free from slime; scales that are tight to the skin, bright and shiny; and flesh that is firm and elastic—it springs back when pressed. The odor is fresh (Walczak, 1977).

Tuna, salmon, mackerel and sardines are good buys in canned fish. Look for cans that have a crimped top seam and no bottom seam. Old-fashioned cans have seams that are soldered with lead. The lead leaches into the contents of the can which results in canned food being our major source of lead poisoning. The FDA has outlawed these cans, so eventually all cans on the market will contain no lead. Tuna is best if water-packed, but some brands have such large amounts of salt added that they're objectionable to the taste. To cut down on the amount of oil, strain the fish and discard the oil. Blot the fish with paper towels.

Sardines are "the cheapest source of high quality protein," says Consumers Union. However, they're high in sodium.

Fresh fish is a better buy than frozen because frozen fish usually loses juices when it thaws. Frozen fish should be cooked before it thaws completely, using any of the recipes in this book.

PREPARATION

There are basically four ways to cook fish: broiling, baking, frying and steaming. Usually large fish are baked, small ones are fried, and fillets and steaks are broiled or sautéed. It takes ten minutes to broil a fish fillet; thirty minutes to bake a whole fish.

In planning a fish meal, let the cut of fish determine your method of cooking, then find a sauce you like. Cook the fish in the sauce or pour the sauce over the fish (Davis, 1947).

The differences in recipes are mainly different sauces. Most of the sauces are rich in fat because most fish have very little fat.

The length of time to cook fish is not set by the pound as it is in meat, but by the thickness. It should be cooked very little. Fish should be flaky but not dry. If fish is salted before it is cooked, the salt draws out the juices, and the flavor is ruined. If fish is coated with crumbs or batter, it may be salted first because the coating catches the delicate juices. Other seasonings than salt should be added before the fish is cooked; since it takes such a short time to cook fish, the flavors should have time to mingle. Most important of all, fish should not be cooked to a higher internal temperature than 150 degrees F because the proteins will get too hard, and the fish will be tough. Besides, it will smell all over the house (Davis, 1947).

Tests for doneness include curling or flaking, but these signs show that the fish is already too done. Stewing fish soaks out flavor, and fish should not be stewed unless they are stewed in the sauce they will be eaten with. Since moist heat cooks faster than dry, it is difficult to steam or stew fish without overcooking it. However, fish may be lightly steamed first then frozen and served later as an appetizer or in salad.

To brown fish, coat it with paprika and crumbs, flour or batter. If the fish is spread with butter then roasted or broiled, it will be delicately browned because the butter browns fast, before the fish is overcooked. The fish may also be "frizzled" which is my word for "fry." Fry means cooking in a hot skillet with hot oil; but heat harms the molecules of oil. Frizzle means cooking in a moderate skillet with butter, which results in molecules that are healthful for our bodies.

POULTRY

PURCHASING

Supermarket and fast-food chickens are raised so poorly that we shouldn't eat them. We can get our chickens from the health food store or from a farmer in the area who raises chickens for his own family and friends. The chickens cost more, but if that is a problem, use chicken as a condiment. At a chicken meal, also serve a cottage cheese salad or tofu, or choose from many other good sources of protein to get your quota.

Almost all supermarket chickens are soaked in water before being shipped. Some of the water is absorbed into the bird, which makes it heavier. You pay more for the water. When the chicken thaws, the water seeps out, and the chicken loses vitamins, minerals, and flavor (Goldbeck, 1973).

Since 1950, arsenic has been used to make 90 percent of all commercial chickens mature early and produce more eggs. It also gives them a deep yellow skin color. Housewives are said to demand the yellow color because they think the chickens are fat and tender. Farmers are supposed to stop giving arsenic before slaughter so it will leave the tissues. But it is known that dangerous amounts are left in the livers when we buy them (Hunter, 1971).

So many antibiotics are used to try to keep chickens from getting infections that fungus and molds grow in their intestines. Birds can gain more weight when given antibiotics, and the chicken houses can be unsanitary without causing thousands of birds to get infectious diseases. This way, as many as 100,000 birds can be kept crowded together with about ¾ of a square foot of space for each (Hunter, 1971).

We don't get turkeys from supermarkets, either; just from the health food store. Commercial turkeys that are self-basting have fat, not necessarily butter, injected into them. The fat, often coconut oil and water, comes to the surface as the turkey cooks, and bastes the turkey. But the cost is high for what you get. Besides, many good cooks say basting just washes nutrients into the gravy. Try unbasted turkey. Turkeys made into turkey rolls usually have too many additives to be healthful (Goldbeck, 1973).

Poultry can be contaminated in any kitchen. Salmonellosis is a very common disease caused by infected animals, including poultry brought home to be cooked. Chickens pick up the germs when put through a water bath in the slaughter house. The germs are destroyed by heat, but when you put a raw chicken on the kitchen counter, it leaves germs that contaminate the cooked chicken and other foods.

Symptoms of salmonellosis are 100 degree fever, diarrhea, vomiting, abdominal cramps and lack of appetite. This lasts two to three days, then it takes several more days before the patient feels really well. The disease can be severe. The best protection is healthy intestinal bacteria, which means that we need to eat yogurt. If antibiotics have been taken, the friendly bacteria may have been destroyed. Thus the patient could easily get Salmonellosis. This ailment looks and acts like the three-day colds and flu that many people, especially children, often have.

PREPARATION

When you get ready to thaw your poultry, put it in the fridge for one or two days. A turkey over eighteen pounds may take three days. If you need to use it sooner, put the bird in its water-tight wrapper in cold water, not in the fridge. Change the water often, and it will thaw faster. Small birds take about an hour; large ones, six to eight hours (Goldbeck, 1973). You can thaw poultry at room temperature, but watch it carefully and cook it when it just becomes pliable.

There are many ways to prepare chicken without using package mixes or other short cuts that destroy food value. Make your own shake-up mixture easily from the recipe on p. 47, Your Own Oven-Fried Chicken.

Turkey should be roasted breast down in a V-shaped rack at a temperature of 300 degrees F the first hour, and 185 F till done—six hours or more, according to size. You can cook a big one overnight.

Choose your poultry from a health food store for better food value and for unbelievably good flavor.

MILK

FRESH MILK

Certified raw milk is said to be the best value of all foods (Walczak, 1977) but selling raw milk is against the law in many areas. Since pasteurized, homogenized milk has been so tampered with by man, let's limit the intake for adults to two glasses a day, one of them yogurt. If you don't have the enzyme (lactase) to digest milk sugar (lactose), you won't be able to drink that much, but you may be able to tolerate some yogurt. Most white Americans have the enzyme; most black Americans don't. If you don't, you'll get abdominal cramps and gas after drinking milk.

Children and teenagers may need more than two glasses, since milk is usually a good source of protein, but it is important to eat plenty of whole grains, legumes, vegetables and whole fruits before filling up on milk.

When milk is pasteurized, as much as 6 percent of the calcium, 20 percent of the total iodine, 9 to 16 percent of the B2 and 25 percent of the B1 are lost (Walczak, 1977). Fifty percent of the vitamin C content is also lost. The cows of this country produce as much vitamin C in one day as the entire crop of citrus fruits in one year, but much of it is lost in pasteurization. Also, all the enzymes in milk are either totally lost or greatly reduced in number (Walczak, 1977).

The growth-promoting hormone in milk is destroyed when milk is pasteurized. Although the food value of pasteurized milk is reduced, it still has enough value to be used as food, if we drink it in moderation, especially if we can't get raw milk. It contains good minerals, vitamins and amino acids, but it is low in iron (Williams, 1971).

When we drink milk, we should drink whole milk because we need fat to assimilate the calcium. However, if we eat too much fat, the calcium and fat form insoluble soaps, and we can't assimilate the calcium. Cream contains chromium, part of the glucose tolerance factor (GTF), which helps keep our blood sugar from being too high or too low. It is highly likely that the last twenty or thirty years of not drinking cream has had something to do with the fact that more and more people have hypoglycemia and diabetes every year.

SOURED MILKS

One of the best forms of milk is yogurt. Buy yours at the health food store or at the few supermarkets that have yogurt made with live culture. This means that the bacteria used as culture were added after the milk was pasteurized and the live bacteria were not killed in pasteurization. You'll see that when you dip a spoon in the yogurt to serve it, a yellowish liquid collects in the hollow. This liquid is whey and has friendly bacteria in it, so be sure to drink it. Also, don't buy the kind with sweetened fruit added. Add your own fresh fruit.

Many people who can't tolerate milk can tolerate yogurt, buttermilk or kefir. We should drink one of these soured milks often—small amounts are all right, up to a cup a day; they're important for the health of the microorganisms in our intestines. Buttermilk isn't as good for our intestinal bacteria as yogurt is.

There are many good recipes for yogurt (see p. 51). Here are a few "recipes" for a yogurt maker.

Get a cardboard carton large enough for a heating pad to lie flat. Place covered jars of yogurt on the pad. Tuck a doubled bath towel around the jars. Cover the box and plug in the heating pad to "medium." Allow about ten hours for a new culture, about three hours to make yogurt from part of the preceding batch.

A nutrition student in my class told me about using a long extension cord with a 25 or 40 watt bulb on the end of it, depending on the size of the oven. That's the easiest of all—just put the bulb in the oven, close the door on the cord, and you can make as many jars as the oven will hold, but don't make more than your family can eat in one week, because the yogurt gets too tart when it gets old. I never can remember to come back and turn off the oven, so I use one of the automatic timers that turn the lights on and off when no one is at home. I set the timer for three hours. Then if I forget, the yogurt doesn't cook so long that it gets too tart.

BUTTERMILK

Buttermilk is good value for your dollar—better than any meat (Walczak, 1977). It's 2 percent butterfat, which is at least better than skimmed milk (Davis, 1947). Most buttermilk on the market is cultured—that is, a small amount of buttermilk, with its lactic acid bacteria which make it sour, is added to skimmed milk or 2 percent fat milk. As the bacteria grow in the new milk, the whole batch becomes sour.

It is very easy to make your own buttermilk. Use 3 ½ cups of milk to one half cup of commercial buttermilk. After 10 or 12 hours at room temperature (about 80 degrees F), the batch is ready; the milk should be stirred well and refrigerated. Use whole milk for the extra nutrients in its cream.

Cultured buttermilk contains more protein, calcium and vitamin B2 than churned buttermilk, so it's more healthful (Davis, 1947).

DRIED MILK

Milk is dried in two ways; one is spray drying, which is how non-instant powdered milk is made. Very little food value is destroyed. The fat is removed, and the rest is pasteurized and partly dried. Then it's blown through nozzles into a vacuum at lower temperatures. This kind of drying doesn't destroy lysine, one of the amino acids (Hunter, 1971).

The other process requires very high heat, which destroys the protein pattern. Large amounts of lysine are lost. The content of vitamin C and of all other vitamins is reduced. Labels at supermarkets may not say which drying process is used, but the instant variety, which dissolves easily in water, is the one processed with high heat. Non-instant powdered milk from the health food store doesn't dissolve easily in water, but it has more food value.

CANNED MILK

Canned evaporated milk loses half its vitamin B6 because of heat in the canning process. There are many additives in canned milk, none of value to health (Gerras, 1972). Sweetened condensed milk is the worst of the canned milks because of the large amount of sugar.

CAROB-FLAVORED MILK

We should never buy chocolate milk. Laboratory experiments show that animals that drink chocolate milk absorb less calcium than those which drink plain milk.

A super form of chocolate-flavored milk is made from carob powder, which looks and tastes like cocoa. It has much less fat, is a high quality carbohydrate and is rather sweet. Any milk drink, pudding or custard flavored with carob is definitely a plus in the diet.

PREPARATION

Milk is ready to drink as is. But many drinks, soups, sauces, desserts and even main dishes can be made with milk.

When you cook milk, use low heat and watch it carefully. If you're making cream soup, heat the milk first, add any acid foods gradually, reheat, and serve as soon as possible. The milk may separate because of the acids, but the soup will taste good.

Dried milk is not a whole food, so it should not be used as one. But it can be added to baked goods and even to whole milk in small amounts to increase the protein content. Every time you use dried milk, use a little soy powder with it to replace lysine (an essential amino acid) which is destroyed in processing the milk. After it is opened, dried milk should be kept in a cool place, tightly covered.

Yogurt can be made at home by adding either yogurt culture or already-prepared yogurt to liquid milk. It's easiest to make yogurt in a yogurt maker. The yogurt should not be moved until it gets thick. Then it should be quickly chilled to stop the growth of the bacteria. If the bacteria continue to grow, the yogurt may get too acid. We shouldn't cook with yogurt because its bacteria are destroyed by heat, and we lose the value of the yogurt.

CREAM

We should buy real cream to whip rather than buying ready-whipped non-dairy products. People usually buy non-dairy products to avoid saturated fat, but the products are made with coconut oil and palm oil, which are highly saturated. These oils are not dangerous in their natural forms, but all the processing and the chemicals in these artificial creams are the reason why they are not recommended (Goldbeck, 1973).

Sour cream is cream that is cultured with bacteria and treated with high heat and pressure, which destroy much of the food value. Homemade yogurt can often take the place of these highly processed dairy products.

CHEESE

Cheese is a good protein food if it's natural and light colored. We don't eat processed cheeses or "cheese foods." Cheese is not constipating or hard to digest, although people think it is. It does take longer to leave the stomach than some foods because the protein is digested there, and fat slows down digestion, but this is natural—it causes no problem.

Natural cheeses usually say "natural" on the label. If you buy from a wheel of cheese in a delicatessen, it will usually be natural. But the test for natural cheese is said to be to ask the clerk for a sliver of cheese. Fold it, and if it's natural, it will crack at the fold.

Light-colored cheeses are best because the dark orange cheeses have too much dye in them. Some good varieties are Swiss, mozzarella and Monterey Jack. There are more and more cheeses being made without the dark colorings—Colby cheddar, among others. These may be available at supermarkets and cheese stores. Excellent cheese is always available at health food stores.

Cheese has few calories compared to its protein value. One ounce of hard cheese supplies about 100 calories. That's about 7.5 percent protein for each calorie. Lean hamburger has about 13 percent protein for each calorie, but bacon and ham have only about 5 percent protein for each calorie. Uncreamed cottage cheese is 19 percent protein per calorie.

The differences in natural and processed cheese make natural a much better buy. Natural cheese may be from a cow, a goat or a sheep, and it is usually whole milk. Sometimes additives are present such as calcium salts, acids, artificial colors and preservatives. Preservatives must be stated on the label, but other additives may not be listed (Goldbeck, 1973).

Processed cheeses are supposedly manufactured so the housewife can melt them more easily. They contain many chemicals and are not as rich as natural cheeses. Pasteurized process cheeses are partly natural, with much water and emulsifiers, plus many chemicals which add texture, color and flavor. Products called "cheese food" have even more chemicals and water. If the label says "spread," there is still more of both. American cheese may have only the word "American" on the label, but that doesn't help much; there is no such thing as natural American cheese (Goldbeck, 1973).

In buying soft cheeses such as cottage cheese, we're getting fresh or dried skim milk, salt and a form of bacteria that causes the curdling. If the cheese is curdled by other acids such as hydrochloric acid or phosphoric acid, we shouldn't eat them. Labels don't have to state these additives or many of the others.

Cream cheese is not a high protein dish—it is a high fat dish. The main additive to avoid is propylene glycol alginate. The rubbery texture of cheese is from vegetable gum or gelatin. Pot cheese is similar to cottage cheese. It is drier, salt-free, and doesn't have additives. Farmer cheese is like cottage and pot cheese, but it is pressed into block form. Most brands contain preservatives. Ricotta cheese is like cottage cheese, but the texture is finer and lighter. It is made from whole or partially skimmed milk. Some brands have many additives which are unnecessary. Feta cheese is sold in a concentrated salt solution. It is sharp and salty—good for salads. All brands have no chemicals.

Mozzarella is a popular cheese—it keeps a little longer than the soft cheeses. There are usually no additives; however some mozzarella that isn't very moist can have preservatives added.

Cheddar, a hard cheese, may have a mold inhibitor added. If so, it will be noted on the label. Pale yellow Swiss cheese may be made of bleached, partially skimmed milk. A number of chemicals can be used. The label will tell you if the milk is treated or if mold inhibitor is used, but if color is added, it doesn't have to be on the label.

Danish cheeses are the least likely to have additives.

If the cheese is labeled, the name of the cheese (if natural) appears alone—e.g., "cheddar cheese"—or is preceded by the word "natural." If the cheese is processed, it will have the words "pasteurized process," "pasteurized process cheese food," or "pasteurized process cheese spread" on the label (Goldbeck, 1973).

PREPARATION

In preparing cheese, cook at low temperatures. In making sauces or other hot foods, add cheese just before serving. Cheese can be melted under the broiler, but it shouldn't brown. The heat must be kept low so the protein won't get tough and stringy.

Many cheese books say to keep cheese wrapped in plastic in the fridge. Mine always gets moldy before we can eat it, so I always grate the cheese (usually in the processor) as soon as I get home with it, then keep it in the freezer. If it's in a block or in slices, it's frozen too hard to use, but I can easily get out part of the grated cheese, use it in a recipe or on toast, without waiting for it to thaw. Cheese dishes should be covered when they are being cooked and served.

Cheese can be added to many dishes, especially if it's grated. Try various kinds and add to soups, salads and egg dishes. It's especially tasty and nutritious on vegetables; it furnishes a good quality protein, and you don't have to use so much butter. Butter is good in moderate amounts, but cheese has more protein.

Since the cheese is high in protein and fat, a small amount satisfies the appetite. Thus a little bit goes a long way.

Most natural cheese is richer in protein than meat, fish or poultry. It is a good source of vitamins A, D, E and B2.

EGGS

Eggs are a near-perfect food. We've been told for the last twenty to thirty years not to eat them because many physicians thought their cholesterol content caused fatty deposits in the arteries. That myth has now been exploded, and it is known that the cholesterol in eggs is balanced by the lecithin in eggs, which keeps fat from stacking up in the blood vessels. It is now known that there are several kinds of cholesterol. The one that the body needs, called HDL (high density lipoprotein) helps transport cholesterol from the tissues to the liver for excretion as bile. This process occurs with the help of an enzyme containing lecithin. Lecithin emulsifies the hard, fatty cholesterol and melts it so it flows through the blood vessels rather than stacking up as hard fat. B vitamins and vitamin C also help keep our cholesterol from stacking up in the arteries.

Of course, it's important not to eat too many eggs, as it is not to eat too much of any one thing. One or two a day are suggested, and more can be used in cooking.

Barnyard eggs have more value than battery (cage) eggs, but even battery eggs have more value than most other common foods (Williams, 1973). We should buy Grade AA and A eggs, either brown or white. The color of the shell has nothing to do with the flavor or nutritive value of the egg (Walczak, 1977).

Buy eggs from the health food store or from a farmer you know whose hens scratch around on the ground. These yard eggs taste so much better, you'll never want to go back to eating cage eggs. Cage eggs have so little flavor that advertisers now resort to saying that "the public demands mild-flavored eggs." They realize the eggs have no flavor, so they're trying to fool us into thinking we like them.

When an egg is broken for cooking, if the yolk looks flat or contains blood spots or mottling, or the white is runny, the egg is probably not fresh (Hunter, 1971).

Eggs kept at room temperature lose more nutrients in one day than those under refrigeration lose in a week. So buy from refrigerated cases and refrigerate immediately when you get them home (Goldbeck, 1973). You can test the freshness yourself. The air pocket inside gets larger as the egg gets older, and therefore a really fresh egg will sink; an old egg will float.

PREPARATION

Many nutritionists say that poached or soft-boiled eggs are best, but there is some controversy about that. They are probably thought best because eggs cooked in those ways are not overcooked (Walczak, 1977). Protein of any kind that is overcooked is harder to digest than protein moderately cooked.

Others say that poached and soft-boiled eggs leave the stomach so fast that almost no digestion can take place, thus few nutrients reach the blood; whereas hard-boiled eggs stay in the stomach until their proteins are digested to liquid (Davis, 1947).

What seems the most sensible idea is to vary our preparation of eggs and depend on a healthy digestive system to digest all good foods.

For the last fifteen or more years, it has been thought that a substance in raw egg whites, called avidin, destroys biotin (a B vitamin) if they are in the digestive tract at the same time. Now many researchers say that raw egg whites are safe to eat, and that the study that showed they weren't was made with rats which were given nothing but raw egg whites. There is enough biotin in the yolk to counteract the avidin, so if we eat both yolk and white, the egg will be healthful. However, another investigator says that raw egg white is indigestible and might cause allergies (Walczak, 1977).

Dr. Steven Cordas (Nutrition Education Conference, Houston, Texas, April 12, 1981) says that raw eggs seem to help many health problems so much that they may contain nutrients that have not been discovered yet. He suggests that raw eggs be used in milk shakes with brewer's yeast for extra nutrients.

To sum up this information about eggs, let's not eat eggs raw if they cause allergies, but let's get rid of our allergies so we can eat anything. (See Allergies and Nutrition, Lesson 4 of A Home Study Course in the New Nutrition.) And let's not eat raw egg whites unless we eat the yolks also.

When you scramble eggs in fat, use butter at a moderate temperature. Don't use margarine or hard white shortening. Both of those fats have high melting points. If we eat fats that melt at our body temperature, they won't stack up in our blood vessels and cause fatty plaques (arteriosclerosis). The fat will melt and flow through the blood vessels.

Eggs should be kept in covered containers in the fridge. Storing eggs with the large end up keeps the yolks centered if you're planning to stuff eggs.

Extra egg whites can be stored in the fridge for a week if tightly covered. If to be kept longer, put them in the freezer. They will keep six months. Yolks should be covered with water and kept in a closed container in the fridge but only for two to three days. They shouldn't be frozen (Goldbeck, 1973).

Prepare beaten egg dishes (omelets or scrambled eggs) by starting them in a moderately hot pan so they won't stick, then moving the pan to a burner already at a lower temperature.

Eggs can be separated more easily when they're cold. Egg whites beat higher when they're at room temperature.

It is hard to tell a cage egg from a yard egg. Cage eggs may have faint black lines circling the shell caused by the egg rolling along the wire base of the cage. I have noticed those lines now that I look for them.

The color of the yolk depends on the hen's diet. Eggs are about 12 percent protein, 12 percent fat (almost all in the yolk), and 74 percent water, with 90 calories in a two-ounce egg. They are a good source of vitamins A and D.

Eggs will stay fresh for three weeks in a fridge, and up to nine months in commercial cold storage. The nutritional value does not deteriorate at these ages, but texture and flavor do. A soft boiled egg white will be milky on the day the egg is laid. It will not whip till it is three days old, and when hard boiled, it will not set firmly till it's a week old (Ballentine, 1978). When you break open an egg, the yolk of a fresh one stays in the center of the white; the yolk of an old one breaks as it leaves the shell.

Fish and skim milk substitute for eggs in commercial baking, and animal blood plasma is used instead of egg whites. Food technologists can spray-dry blood plasma, mix it with locust bean kernel, and have it come out like egg white. This would look good on a lemon meringue pie, but it might be rather traumatic to think you're eating blood protein (Seddon and Burrow, 1977).

LIQUID PROTEIN

Liquid protein is not a good source of protein if it's made of collagen, the tough, fibrous connective tissue (tendons, ligaments, etc). These parts are usually liquefied to make gelatin. They can be processed down to amino acids, but they do not have enough methionine, one of the essential amino acids needed to make a complete protein. Body protein has to be broken down to supply the methionine. Most of that incomplete protein is of the lowest quality and is the least suitable for the body (Ballentine, 1978).

RECIPES

MUSCLE MEATS

In basic cooking of meats such as roasting, frying, etc., the most important point to remember is not to overcook protein, because the body can't digest it. Most recipes emphasize that the meat should be seared at moderately high temperatures to destroy the surface bacteria, then turned to low to finish cooking.

Most health food cookbooks have many good recipes for animal proteins. Other cookbooks may use canned meats, soups, or other processed foods in combination with animal protein dishes such as stews, loaves, and others. The processed "additives" don't have the food value found in binders such as eggs, wheat germ, powdered milk, soy powder or leftover cooked whole grains. They can be enriched with ground seeds or soy grits soaked in hot water for five minutes before mixing with other ingredients.

COMBO STEAK

This steak will surprise you with its tangy flavor. It's a combination of round steak and yogurt. Cut into 4 serving size pieces and dredge with wholewheat flour:

1 pound round steak, fat trimmed off

Melt in skillet:
1 T butter
Brown steak on both sides in butter
Add:
3 T water
½ t paprika
1 sliced onion
½ c yogurt
1½ T grated Swiss or light-colored, natural
cheddar cheese
Cover skillet and simmer about 2 to 3 hours
(depending on thickness) or until meat is tender.
Yield: 4 servings

MEAT LOAF

Preheat oven to 325 F. Mix and soak for two
minutes:
½ c soy grits
2 T food yeast (optional)
1 c milk
Chop by hand or in processor:
1 onion
1 clove garlic
1 rib celery cut in chunks
2 carrots cut in chunks
2 sprigs parsley
¼ c pumpkin seeds
Mix soy and vegetables in large bowl with:
1 pound lean ground beef
1 egg
1½ t salt
½ t sage
Pack in buttered loaf pan. Bake 1 hour. Remove from pan immediately so the grease won't
soak back into the meat.
Yield: 6 servings

HAMBURGERS FOR HEALTH

Grate by hand or in processor (steel blade):
two 1″ cubes of cheese
1 rib celery
1 onion cut in chunks
3 to 4 sprigs of parsley
1 carrot cut in chunks
Mix in bowl with:
1 pound lean ground beef
2 eggs
1 t sea salt
2 T food yeast (optional)

Form into patties, pan broil in butter.
Yield: 6 servings

QUICKIE CABBAGE LEAVES AND BEEF

Core and pull leaves apart:
1 medium size head of cabbage
Steam until the leaves have wilted. Preheat
oven to 350 F. Chop in processor:
1½ c drained, pitted ripe olives
Combine with olives and mix well:
1½ pounds ground beef round
¼ c finely chopped onion
1 egg, lightly beaten
¼ t black pepper (optional)
½ c soft wholewheat bread crumbs or wheat
germ
¼ c milk
½ t caraway seeds
¼ t thyme
Line a buttered 9×5×3×″ pan with cabbage
leaves. Cover with half the meat. Add another
layer of cabbage leaves and top with more meat
and another layer of cabbage leaves. Cover
loosely with aluminum foil, place on a baking
sheet and bake 1¼ hours. Remove foil. Hold
wire cooling rack over loaf and drain off liquid
into a measuring cup.
Reserve. Serve with:
cream sauce flavored with white wine or beef
broth.
Yield: 6–8 servings

BEEF AND VEGETABLE MAIN DISH

Frizzle in a large skillet which has a cover:
1 pound ground meat sprinkled with sea salt
When brown, turn out on paper towels and
scrub some of the fat off. Return to skillet and
add:
1 medium onion
1½ c your choice of vegetables, such as
squash, potatoes, carrots, cabbage, green
beans, or a mixture of several
few sprigs of parsley
½ c leftover beans or grains (optional)
vegetable powder seasoning
Cover with lid, cook until tender, not mushy.
Serve over brown rice or other grain or biscuits.
Yield: 6–8 servings

VEGETABLE-MEAT CASSEROLE

Set oven at 350 F. Steam till slightly tender:
    2 large zucchini cut in ½″ slices (not peeled)
    2 c home-frozen tomatoes, peeled
    1 large onion, sliced thin
    2 large green peppers, sliced
    2 large carrots, sliced thin
Frizzle in moderate skillet till meat loses its pink color:
    1 pound lean ground meat
Arrange meat and vegetables in layers in casserole. Sprinkle each layer with vegetable broth powder and a little salt. Bake in oven for 1 hour. Pour over the mixture:
    4 eggs slightly beaten
Cover, cook in oven for 15 more minutes. Serve with brown rice or millet or over chunky slices of whole wheat toast. If there are leftovers, cut into squares, wrap and freeze. Warm in toaster oven at 300 F, or in steamer with brown rice for a complete meal.

In preparing any ground meat dish like this, drain the fat off the meat, pour the cooked meat out onto heavy paper towels, and scrub it to get as much grease off as possible.
Yield: 6–8 servings

MEATBALLS

Mix well, form into walnut-sized balls:
    2 pounds lean ground beef
    2 eggs
    1 t vegetable salt
    2 T wheat bran
    ½ c milk
    2 t wheat germ
Place balls on a grill or on a rack over a broiler pan. Bake in oven at 375 F for about 15 minutes.
Yield: 6–8 servings

SOUP STOCK

To make soup stock with meat, cook soup bones in water with vinegar in it to help draw the calcium out of the bones and into the soup. Add salt to help draw out juices from the soup meat. Remove marrow from the bones and stir it into the stock. Make soup stock the day before you make the soup. Refrigerate so the fat will rise to the top; skim it off and throw it away.

HAMBURGER PIZZA

We make pizza that is delicious and healthful. While you may have thought it's a lot of trouble to make, here's a quickie method.

First make the crust.
Place in a small bowl and let stand till foamy:
    ¼ c warm water (not hot)
    1 T dry brewer's yeast
In the large bowl of your mixer:
    2 c hot tap water
    ½ T sugar
    ½ T salt
    3 c wholewheat flour
Mix till smooth. Add yeast. Mix, adding:
    2 c flour (approximately)
Mix until stretchy. The dough will change before your eyes. Roll and pat out, stretching gently to a size about 2 inches larger than your buttered pizza pan. Let rest while making sauce.

Mix in blender or processor (plastic blade):
    1 c peeled home-frozen or fresh tomatoes
    ½ t vinegar
    1 small clove garlic (optional)
    ½ t pizza seasoning
    ½ t flaked oregano
    ½ c dry cottage cheese (optional)
Pour the sauce on the crust. Grate cheese by hand or in a processor and spread over sauce. Add ½ pound of frizzled hamburger meat scrubbed between paper towels to get the grease out. Add steamed or chopped green pepper or other vegetable. Bake at 350 F about 20 minutes. If you freeze all or part of the pizza, you may prefer to add grated cheese when reheating it. I cut the pieces to fit my toaster-oven tray and wrap and freeze them.
Yield: 2 12″ pizzas

CHILI

Heat in a heavy skillet:
  3 T butter
Sauté in butter until tender:
  1 small onion, chopped fine
  1 small green pepper, chopped
In separate skillet, brown and stir till the meat loses its pink color:
  1½ pounds lean ground meat
Pour the meat into a colander to drain out the fat. Discard the fat. Pour the meat on heavy paper towels and "scrub" to get more fat out. Return the meat to the pan with onion and pepper. Add, stir, cover and cook over low heat for an hour:
  2 T chili powder or to taste
  1 t sea or vegetable salt
  2 c peeled home-frozen, canned or fresh tomatoes
    or 1 c homemade tomato sauce
Store in fridge or freezer.
Yield: 6–8 servings

ORGAN MEATS

Calves' liver is an organ meat that is acceptable. Although the liver is an animal's detoxifying organ, the toxins are not stored in the liver. They're stored in the fat cells and in the lining of the intestines, to be excreted. Many restaurants and cafeterias serve liver every day. This is a good choice when you eat out.

LIVER AND APPLES

Yes, not Liver and Onions, but Liver and Apples. Sounds good for a change, doesn't it?

Cut into noodle-like strips, using a sharp knife or a large pair of scissors:
  Lamb or calves' liver
Sauté in a heavy skillet in butter until golden brown:
  sliced apples
Add the liver to the apples in the skillet, toss, and sauté for another three minutes. Season with vegetable salt and powdered vegetable seasoning.
Yield: 4–6 servings

LIVER 'N' PEACHES

Turn on both sides to coat:
  1 lb. liver slices
  wheat germ
Frizzle in heavy skillet in butter for about five minutes. Add and simmer three to five minutes longer:
  2 T chopped onion
  2 T tomatoes, chopped
Add and heat until warmed through:
  2 fresh ripe or home-frozen peaches, sliced

If you're freezing peaches for smoothies, here's a new way to use your home-frozen peaches.
Yield: 4–6 servings

SPECIAL LIVER

Melt in skillet:
  2 T butter
Add and sauté till lightly browned:
  1 T chopped onion
Add and brown on both sides then reduce heat and cook five minutes:
  4 thin slices calves' liver
Remove meat and arrange on heated serving plate. Add to pan drippings and stir one minute:
  ⅓ c dry red wine
    or 1 apple, chopped
Pour gravy over liver.
Yield: 4 servings

FROZEN RAW LIVER

Freeze raw liver or brains. Grate and add to tomato juice; drink immediately. Infants love this (Walczak, 1977).

A delightful fringe benefit of my letter for permission to use Dr. Walczak's suggestion for raw liver juice for babies was a personal note from Mrs. Alberta Stone, Executive Secretary of the International College of Applied Nutrition, publisher of the booklet *Nutrition Applied Personally,* in which the raw liver juice recipe was published.

Mrs. Stone wrote: "Yes, you certainly may use the Frozen Raw Liver suggestion. We would hope a lot more people get the information, it really does do a lot of good.

"If I may get personal—Dr. Pottenger put me

on three 'liver cocktails' per day for a while, following testing showing I had pernicious anemia. That was approximately 40 years ago. And to date no evidence of any type of anemia is found in my blood check-ups.

"Also, when our second child was born (in 1945), she was not anemic, as I had been drinking 'raw blood' Dr. Pottenger supplied me with during the pregnancy. (He was doing this experimentally then.) The baby's blood was exactly twice as good as mine. However, he still had me give her, at age two weeks and on, raw frozen liver. I grated about one teaspoonful, put it in a spoon over warm water (to remove the chill), then put that in her mouth followed by her bottle (unfortunately I was never able to produce milk). After she got her first teeth, he had me give her beef and brains, prepared the same way."

FRIZZLED LIVER

Dredge 4 slices liver in salted oat flour; frizzle in a little butter over moderate heat.
Yield: 4 servings

TALK-SHOW LIVER

Sometimes it pays to listen to talk shows. I heard this recipe on a talk show, and I was glad I was listening.

Spread salad mustard on one side of 4 liver slices. Turn slice over in a bowl of wheat germ. Spread the other side with mustard; turn again to coat with wheat germ. Cook slowly in dry skillet, about 15 minutes each side. This is good to freeze and eat cold for lunch or in a sandwich, because there's no taste of cold grease.
Yield: 4 servings

SWEETBREADS

Soak 1 lb. sweetbreads in cold water with 1 T vinegar for ½ hour. Parboil gently for 20 minutes; remove membranes when cool. Cut into bite size, serve diced with hard boiled egg in white sauce over toast.
Yield: 4–6 servings

FISH

I always tell people "Eat all the fish you want." That's a broad statement when I also say, "Vary your diet." But I haven't found anyone who wanted to eat fish twice every day. Five to seven times a week would be all right, because man doesn't do much to fish except catch, package and ship it. We can eat frozen fish, fresh fish of course, and even canned tuna, salmon and sardines—not as good as the fish you catch yourself, but acceptable. Halibut is a good, small ocean fish, which shouldn't be polluted as much as the larger fish at the top of the food chain.

BROILED FISH

Combine in a bowl and mix well:
  ½ c cornmeal
  1 t salt
Dip in the mixture:
  1 pound fish fillets
Arrange fillets in an oiled shallow pan lined with foil—dull side next to food. Put them at least 6 inches from the broiler so they brown slowly; cook from six to ten minutes on each side, depending on thickness.
Yield: 3 servings

FISH BAKED IN SAUCE

Prepare in blender one or two cups of medium cream sauce; add 1 t fennel seeds, cheese, dill or other seasoning. Place sauce in baking dish; add 4 fish fillets or steaks. Spoon some sauce over fish and sprinkle on top:
  wheat germ or bread crumbs
  paprika
Bake at 300 F about 10 minutes for ½-inch thick fillets, or till done. Garnish with:
  parsley
  lemon wedges
Yield: 4 servings

OVEN-FRIED FISH

This recipe surprised me because it is so simple, yet tastes so good, and it doesn't burn at the high temperature. Watch it the first time you try it, especially if the fish slices are thicker or thinner than ½ inch.

Dip 6 serving-size pieces of fresh or barely thawed fish (½ inch thick) in milk. Coat with wheat germ or wholewheat bread crumbs or a mixture of both. Bake in greased pan 10–15 minutes in a 500 F oven. No turning or basting is needed—don't overcook. The fish is juicy and has a nice brown crust. For thicker slices, cook longer and cover pan with foil.
Yield: 6 servings

FILLET FISH ALMONDINE

Choose 6 6-oz. slices of fresh or frozen haddock, perch, flounder or other white fish.
Melt in baking dish:
    ¼ c butter
Dip fillets in butter on both sides, then place skin side down in dish. Sprinkle with paprika and ¼ c finely sliced almonds. Bake in a 400 degree F oven about 15 minutes. Sprinkle with parsley.
Yield: 6 servings

POACHED FISH

Place in saucepan or large skillet and heat about 5 minutes:
    ½ c water
    1 T lemon juice
    1 T vinegar
    sprinkle of thyme, savory or marjoram
Add in 6-oz. pieces and simmer 5–10 minutes until it flakes easily:
    1 pound fish fillets or steaks
Serve leftover fish with yogurt dressing or add it to chowder.
Yield: 3 servings

NEWBURG SPECIAL

Add sherry or white table wine to the sauce when you bake fish.
    1 T of wine per cup of white sauce.

TUNA CHOWDER

Steam:
    1 chopped onion
    2 large potatoes, diced
    1 stalk celery, diced
    1 carrot, diced (optional)

Turn vegetables into pan, add, and heat to simmering;
    2 c fresh milk
    1 t dried vegetable powder or herbs of your choice
    1 t Worcestershire sauce
When vegetables are soft, blend in blender and add:
    1 c milk
    ½ c or so of the steamed potato
    ⅓ c non-instant powdered milk
Return to pan and add:
    2 cans water packed tuna, drained, or other fish or leftover fish. Heat and serve.
Yield: 6–8 servings

FRIZZLED FISH

"Frizzled" means cooked at a moderate temperature in butter. If fish is frozen, allow it to almost thaw. Roll in cornmeal and salt to taste. Place in moderate skillet in butter. Cook till golden brown. Turn and cook other side. This crust is delicious and healthful.

SALMON CROQUETTES

Make cream sauce with:
    3 T butter
    5 T wholewheat flour
    1 c milk
Add:
    1 pound canned salmon, drained
    2 c mashed potatoes
    1½ t salt
    ⅛ t pepper
    1 beaten egg
    1 T minced parsley
    1 t lemon juice
Form into flat shapes such as patties and frizzle until golden brown.
Yield: 6 servings

DEVILED SHRIMP (OR OTHER SEAFOOD)

Make cream sauce (p. 27), add seasonings:
    grated onion
    salt to taste
    dash of cayenne
    1½ c chopped shrimp or other seafood
    ¼ t thyme
    2 T sherry
    2 t salad mustard

Bake 15 to 20 minutes at 350 F in casserole set in hot water. Sprinkle with:

    buttered bread crumbs
    Parmesan cheese (optional)
    paprika

To freeze: Add topping when ready to serve.
Yield: 3 servings

SALMON DIP OR SPREAD

Blend in blender:

    ½ c cottage cheese
    2 T soy sauce
    1 T lemon juice

Add and mix well:

    1 1-lb. can salmon, drained and flaked
    1 8-oz. can water chestnuts, drained and chopped,
    or 1 c chopped Jerusalem artichokes if available
    1 small onion, minced
    1 stalk celery, minced

Serve on toast strips or on split buttered biscuits.
Yield: 6–8 servings

POULTRY

FOWL IS FAIR

Blend in blender till smooth:

    Juice from a small can of chunk pineapple
    1 T arrowroot or cornstarch
    2 T soy sauce
    ⅓ c water

Pour into saucepan, add, and simmer till thick:

    2 c leftover diced turkey or chicken
    chunk pineapple

Heat well and serve on brown rice or cracked wheat.
Yield: 4 servings

YOUR OWN OVEN-FRIED CHICKEN

Here's "fried" chicken without the highly heated oil that makes it dangerous to our health. This is the way to prepare fried chicken that is as healthful as it is tasty.

Preheat oven to 350 F. Beat together in shallow bowl:

    1 egg
    ½ c milk

Combine in paper bag:

    ½ c wholewheat flour
    1 T baking powder
    1 T sea salt
    2 T paprika
    2 T sesame seeds
    1 3-lb. chicken, skinned

Dip chicken in egg mixture and shake in bag. Place the pieces in a baking dish so they don't touch each other. Dot with butter; bake till done, about 1 hour.
Yield: 4–6 servings

CHICKEN AND VEGGIES

Steam:

    1 large white onion, sliced thin
    1 green pepper, sliced thin
    ⅛ t black pepper

Add to steamer and steam until done (about 25 minutes):

    2 large carrots, sliced diagonally
    2 large potatoes, sliced
    2 whole chicken breasts, skinned and cut in bite-size pieces.

Season with a little butter.
Yield: 4 servings

CURRIED CHICKEN OR TURKEY

This recipe is ideal for leftover chicken or turkey.
Heat and simmer:

    2 c stock
    1 T butter (if fowl is dry)

Cut in bite-size pieces, add, and simmer:

    1 large chopped onion
    1 cucumber
    1 apple
    1 sweet potato

Add:

    ¼ c seedless raisins
    1 t to 2 T curry powder

For every cup of stock, place in bowl:

    1 T cornstarch

Moisten cornstarch in a little cold stock. Stir it into the boiling stock. Just before serving, stir in:

1 c cream

Heat the sauce, but do not let it boil. Add 2 c diced chicken and serve the curry over brown rice.

Yield: 4 servings

CHICKEN OR TURKEY A LA KING

Dice and mix together:
    1 c cooked chicken
    ½ c sautéed fresh mushrooms
    ¼ c canned pimentos
Blend together:
    3 T butter
    3 T wholewheat flour
Add slowly:
    1½ c chicken stock, or cream or combination
When sauce is smooth and boiling, add the chicken mixture. Reduce the heat and add:
    1 egg yolk
Stir until the sauce thickens slightly.
Add:
    seasoning to taste
    1 T sherry (optional)
    ¼ c slivered, toasted almonds
Yield: 4 servings

CHICKEN TAMALE PIE

Cook cornmeal mush. Combine and stir:
    ½ c corn meal or grits
    ½ c cold water
    ½ t salt
Place in top of steamer:
    2 c boiling water
Stir in the cornmeal and water slowly. Cook over medium heat for 10 minutes. Steam it covered for 1 hour or more. Stir frequently.

Cut into bite-size pieces:
    3 c cooked chicken
Line a baking dish with the mush. Place the chicken over it. Combine:
    1 c tomato sauce
    1 c corn cut off the cob
    2 T butter, melted
    10 ripe or stuffed olives, sliced
    1 t salt
    pepper to taste
    1 t dried basil or tarragon (optional)

Pour the sauce mixture over the chicken. Sprinkle the top with grated Parmesan cheese. Bake in a 350 F oven about 45 minutes.

Yield: 6 servings

"ANY" CASSEROLE

Mix in large bowl:
    1½ slices wholewheat bread crumbs or left-
       over brown rice
    sprinkle black pepper
    3 beaten egg yolks
    3 c of any of the following:
       canned water-packed tuna
       cooked ground beef
       diced cooked chicken
       well-drained cooked vegetables
    ½ c milk
    2 T butter, melted in dish you'll bake in
    1½ c grated sharp cheese
Fold in:
    3 beaten egg whites
Pour into shallow baking dish set in a pan of boiling water. Bake at 350 F about 30 minutes or till set.

Cut leftovers into serving-size pieces; wrap in foil. Freeze. Later, reheat in steamer or low-temperature toaster oven while still wrapped.

Yield: 6–8 servings

"ANY PATTIES"
Alias
"INSTANT CREPES"

Preheat oven to 350 F. Mix in blender:
    ½ c milk
    2 eggs
    ¼ c wholewheat flour
    ¼ c wheat germ
    ½ t salt
    2 T powdered milk
    2 T soy powder
    1 t baking powder
Pour the mixture over 2 c cooked ground beef, fish, diced chicken, drained vegetables, or any combination. Mix well and spoon onto buttered baking sheet. The liquid shouldn't run; if it does, add a little more flour. Bake about 20 minutes at 350 F. Serve sprinkled with grated cheese or serve with nut milk sauce or fruit

relish. If you're making turkey patties, serve with cranberry sauce.
Yield: 4–6 servings.

Or: (This is faster.) Drop by large spoonfuls onto a lightly buttered, moderately hot skillet, turn and cook other side. Don't cook too brown; allow for extra browning when leftover frozen patties are reheated.

To reheat: Place on the tray of the toaster oven and cover loosely with foil so the top won't burn. Heat at 300 F for about 10 minutes or leave in foil wrap they were frozen in, place in steamer to thaw and heat with vegetables or meat for a complete meal.

Optional seasonings: Chopped dried apricots, dried rosemary, nutmeg, coriander, basil, other favorite spices, or grated Swiss cheese, Parmesan cheese, parsley, or toasted sunflower or sesame seeds.

This is a good, quick prepare-ahead recipe. Mix five times the amounts given of the dry ingredients and store in the freezer. Use ¾ c of dry ingredients, plus two eggs and ½ c milk with two cups of the cooked meat, fish or vegetables, or the combination. I call these patties "Instant Crepes" because they have all the same ingredients as the usual crepes and taste very much the same, but they're quicker to make.

CHEESE DISHES

WELSH RAREBIT

Blend in blender, then heat to simmering, stirring often:
   ¾ c whole milk
   ½ c powdered milk
   ¼ t vegetable or sea salt
   ¾ t dry mustard
   pinch cayenne
   1 t brewer's yeast (optional)
Remove from heat and add:
   ½ pound (2 c) sharp cheese, diced. Stir well, cover pan, let stand 6–8 minutes till cheese is melted; stir again. Serve over toast or vegetables.

Or: Use a blend of cheeses: Swiss, jack, pimento, Roquefort.

Or: Use only Swiss cheese; prepare dry,

toasted wholegrain bread in cubes. Dip cubes into rarebit.
Yield: 6–8 servings

CHEESE FONDUE

Combine 1 c soft wholewheat bread cubes with 1 c fresh milk; add ingredients of Welsh Rarebit without heating, plus 2 eggs beaten separately, and 1 t brewer's yeast (optional). Bake in slow oven for 25 minutes at 325 F.
Yield: 8 servings

CHEESE AND TORTILLAS

Sauté in skillet in butter, mixing the butter well with the tortillas:
   12 tortillas torn into 2″ squares
   1 t chili powder
   ½ t crushed oregano
Blend in blender until smooth:
   1½ c cottage cheese
   1½ c tomato sauce
Pour blender mix over tortilla pieces in skillet, top with:
   ½ pound jack cheese
      (2½ c grated)
Cover skillet and heat through till the cheese is melted and the sauce bubbly.
Yield: 4–6 servings

CHEESE BALLS

Mix together and form into bite-size balls:
   1 8-oz. package Swiss cheese, grated
   ½ c soft butter
   1 t mustard
   1 t Worcestershire sauce
   2 T dry sherry
   dash of tabasco (optional)
   ½ to 1 c finely chopped walnuts
Serve with toothpicks for spearing.
Yield: 18–20 balls

SWISS CHEESE SPREAD OR DIP

Mix well:
   ½ c grated Swiss cheese
   ½ c blended cottage cheese
   ¼ c chopped dill weed
      or 1 t salad mustard to taste

1 T or so of soft butter
pepper to taste
Yield: 4 servings

SHARP WHITE CHEDDAR SPREAD

Combine and mix well:
  1 8-oz. package white cheddar cheese, grated
  ¼ c soft butter
  ¼ to ½ t chili powder
  1 t Worcestershire sauce
  ½ small onion, minced
Serve with Crispy-Chewy Corn Chips or Corn Dodgers.
Yield: 4–6 servings

QUICHE LORRAINE

Set oven at 350 F. Make a wholewheat pastry crust (see p. 113), or line a buttered baking pan or pie pan with thin-sliced whole grain bread.

In blender, beat lightly and pour into pie shell:
  4 eggs
  1 c grated Swiss cheese or Gruyère
  ¼ c Parmesan cheese
  2 c milk
  ¼ t nutmeg
  ⅛ t white pepper
  ½ t sea salt
  ¼ c soy bacon chips
Bake on lower shelf of oven for 45 minutes.
Yield: 4–6 servings

PEANUT QUICHE

Set oven at 375 F. Make a nine-inch whole grain pie crust (see p. 113).

In blender, mix and pour into crust:
  4 eggs
  1 ¾ c whole milk
  2 T chopped green onion
  ¼ t salt
  ¾ c toasted peanuts, chopped
  4 ounces (1 c) Swiss cheese, grated
Bake 45–50 minutes or till just set. Let stand 10 minutes, cut and serve.
Yield: 6–8 servings

CHEESE THE EASY WAY

Cut into ½-inch slices:
  whole grain bread
Spread the slices lightly with:
  butter
Cut two of the slices twice across from corner to corner, making 8 triangular pieces. Cut the rest of the bread into cubes. There will be about four cups of diced, buttered bread. Place layers of cubed bread alternately with layers of:
  1 c grated cheese
Combine and beat:
  2 eggs
  1 c milk
  1 t salt
  ¼ t paprika
  ½ t dry mustard
Pour the egg mixture over the bread and cheese. Place the triangles of bread around the edge of the dish. Bake at 350 F for 20 minutes.
Yield: 6–8 servings

PEPPERS FILLED WITH CHEESE RICE

Prepare 4 green peppers for stuffing. Cut the stem ends from peppers and take out the seeds and veins. Place the peppers in the steamer and cook until they are nearly tender. Drain well. Fill and cover with butter or sprinkle with bread crumbs or cheese.

Mix well:
  1 c cooked rice or other grain
  ½ c stock, cream or tomato pulp
  salt to taste
  paprika
  ½ t curry powder (optional)
  ½ c or more grated cheese
Fill the peppers. Cover the tops with:
  bread crumbs
  butter
  cheese
Put the peppers in the steamer and steam for 10 or 15 minutes, or bake at 350 F for the same length of time.
Yield: 4 servings

COTTAGE CHEESE

You may want to make your own cottage cheese. Use the whey in beverages and soups.

Combine, using wire whisk or blender:
    2 c skim milk powder
    8 c water
Strain to remove lumps. Cover with a cloth; leave at room temperature 1–2 days till sour. Heat very slowly. Test by pressing between thumb and forefinger. When you can hold the curds between your fingers and they don't slip away, pour the milk through a cheesecloth-lined strainer, catching the whey in a bowl. Allow the cheese to drain. Refrigerate both whey and cheese.

Or: To make yogurt cheese, place yogurt in cheesecloth-lined strainer; don't squeeze. Drip overnight in fridge; it's ready to eat.

COTTAGE CHEESE SOUP

Sauté till soft:
    2 T butter
    2 T minced onion
Blend in blender and add to butter and onion:
    4 c milk
    ½ t paprika
    dash of nutmeg
    1 t celery seed
    1 t vegetable salt
    2 c cottage cheese
Heat slightly, do not boil.
Yield: 6 servings

SOURED MILKS

YOGURT

Mix in blender and heat to lukewarm:
    1 quart of whole milk
    2 c non-instant powdered milk
    1 quart of water

Stir in:
    6 ounces yogurt from previous batch or new culture.
Stir well but don't agitate excessively. Pour into jars, cover, and place in yogurt maker. Check consistency at end of three hours. Chill as soon as milk thickens. The first batch made with a new culture usually takes up to ten hours.
Yield: 8 servings

MY FAVORITE YOGURT

This yogurt sets up well, but when you stir it, you can drink it. This is what I take my vitamin and mineral supplement tablets with. Since it's thick, the tablets go down easily.

In blender, blend at low about 1 second:
    2 c warm water
    ½ c previous batch of yogurt
Pour into large bowl.
In blender mix well:
    2 c warm water
    ½ c non-instant powdered milk
Pour into same bowl and add:
    1 quart whole milk
    1 large can evaporated milk
Fill six pint jars and place in yogurt maker.
Yield: 8–10 servings

CONTINUOUS YOGURT

The first time you buy an envelope of yogurt culture or a container of yogurt from the health food store to make your own yogurt from, follow directions on the label or use one of the above recipes. After the yogurt is made, save out about ½ cup. Freeze the rest in ice cube trays. Then release the yogurt cubes and keep in the freezer in a plastic bag. About once a month use 2 or 3 cubes as a new culture. Make yogurt to eat with the ½ cup you held out. You can make yogurt from the preceding batch each week for a month.

7

CHINESE-AMERICAN DISHES

A VISIT TO CHINA

A delightful trip to China and two meals a day for fourteen days of Chinese food inspired these recipes that taste like Chinese foods but are more healthful. They contain no highly heated (and carcinogenic) vegetable oils; rather, they are "frizzled" with butter instead of hot oil. They are made with brown rice and whole grains rather than white rice and white flour. The food is much easier to prepare.

Most of the meals served in China include meat, poultry, seafood or tofu (soybean cheese), cut in small pieces (easy to eat with chopsticks), combined with vegetables, heated in a wok, steamed till tender and served with a tasty sauce.

Usually when the group I traveled with entered a restaurant, the first course was already on the table. It consisted of several kinds of dried meat, seafood and fresh vegetables. We passed the serving plates around the table, helping ourselves with chopsticks.

The next course follows soon after, with six or eight more dishes to come, which the Chinese serve one at a time and call "courses." Usually there are as many courses as there are people to be served, with soup and rice on the menu in addition.

The following ingredients are a part of most Chinese dishes. Also, some more healthful or more available substitutions are suggested for American cooks.

Chinese . . . .*American*
Chinese wine . . . . cooking sherry
soy sauce . . . . .tamari soy sauce
sesame or peanut oil . . . . .butter
white sugar . . . . . . .dark brown sugar or honey
salt .vegetable or sea salt
monosodium glutamate . . . . .omit
cornstarch . . . . .same or arrowroot starch

Occasionally, the recipe will call for additional seasonings and vegetables:

onion   garlic
green pepper   celery
fresh or home-frozen tomatoes
dried powdered ginger or fresh grated ginger
    root
green vegetables

CHINESE MEAT AND VEGETABLES

To prepare the meat, fish or chicken, cut it in bite-size pieces and frizzle it in a skillet with a little butter until brown, then transfer it to the steamer and steam till tender.

To prepare the vegetables, chop or slice them and stir in a large skillet with butter at a moderate temperature for two or three minutes. Set aside.

CHINESE SAUCES

To prepare the sauce, mix the following ingredients:

    1 c chicken stock
    1 t sugar
    ⅛ white pepper (optional)
    1 T wine
    1 T soy sauce
    tomato sauce to taste
    fresh lemon juice to taste (optional)
    2 T cornstarch (optional)

Add the sauce mixture (except for the cornstarch) to the vegetables and simmer for three or four minutes. Mix the cornstarch with a small amount of water, add to the sauce and stir until it thickens slightly. Add the meat (chicken, fish, tofu) and stir well until heated through.

For sweet-sour sauce, add 1 or 2 T vinegar and 1 or 2 T of sugar or honey, depending on your taste.
Yield: 1¼–1½ cups

You see now how these simplified Chinese dishes are made. Use your own preferences and make new combinations for more fun and more taste treats.
To get started, let's use some recipes adapted from typical Chinese dishes.

SWEET-SOUR PORK

Make a batter of:
  2 T wholewheat flour
  ½ t salt
  ⅛ t pepper
  1 egg
Dip in the batter and frizzle in a skillet with butter until a light brown, transfer to steamer and cook till tender:
  1 pound pork cut into cubes.
Add to skillet and simmer for 10 minutes:
  ½ c chicken bouillon
  1 or 2 green peppers, seeded and cut into 1 inch squares
  ½ c pineapple juice
Mix, add to bouillon mixture, and cook until clear:
  an additional ½ c chicken bouillon
  2 T cornstarch
  2 to 4 T vinegar
  2 T soy sauce
  2 to 4 T sugar or honey
Add the pork to the sauce and simmer for five minutes. Serve over hot brown rice.
Yield: 6 servings

CHICKEN AND RICE

Bring to a boil:
  3 c chicken stock

  ¼ c cooking sherry
  ¼ c soy sauce
  1 T honey
Add and cook till celery is done:
  1 pound cooked chicken meat, sliced thin
  2 large stalks celery, thinly sliced at an angle
Add and boil for five minutes:
  3 long green onions, cut in 1″ lengths
Serve hot over cooked brown rice.
Yield: 4–6 servings

SWEET-SOUR FISH

Cut fillets into serving-size pieces and frizzle in butter at moderate heat until golden:
  1 3-pound white fish
Mix well, boil for a few minutes, and pour over fish:
  3 T butter
  1 t cornstarch
  ¼ c apple cider vinegar
  ¼ t powdered ginger
  ⅛ c dark brown sugar
  1 t soy sauce
  1 large onion, chopped fine
Yield: 8 servings

EGG AND MUSHROOM SOUP

Simmer in a wide, shallow saucepan until onions are almost tender:
  2 c chicken stock
  6 T sherry
  6 T soy sauce
  2 onions, sliced thin
Slice thinly, add, and heat through:
  1 cup cooked chicken
  1 cup mushrooms
Beat lightly and add all at once:
  6 eggs
When the eggs are half cooked, quickly pour the soup over six individual bowls of hot brown rice and serve.
Yield: 6 servings

TUNA AND RICE PATTIES

Mix in a bowl:
  2 c cooked brown rice
  1 can tuna fish
  2 eggs

½ small onion, chopped
salt and pepper to taste
¼ to ½ t curry powder
Form into patties and frizzle in a moderate skillet in butter.
Yield: 4 servings

CHICKEN AND WALNUTS

Frizzle in skillet in butter then set aside:
½ c chopped walnuts
Clean, cut in bite-size pieces, and frizzle in butter in large skillet, then transfer to steamer and steam till tender:
½ chicken
Mix well and stir in skillet till slightly thick:
1 T cornstarch
1 t sugar
6 large mushrooms, sliced
2 T soy sauce
1 c water or chicken stock
Stir for five minutes until the mushrooms are tender. Remove from fire, add chicken, and serve over hot brown rice. Sprinkle walnuts on top.
Yield: 6 servings

VEGETABLES AND . . .

Cut in small pieces and frizzle in butter in moderate skillet till well done:
½ pound pork, beef, or chicken
1 onion chopped fine
Transfer meat to steamer. Add and steam until tender:
½ head cabbage cut in 1 inch pieces
3 green peppers cut in 1 inch squares
3 T soy sauce
Add and serve over hot brown rice:
¼ t powdered ginger
1 t sugar
Yield: 6 servings

SHRIMP FOO YUNG

Beat well, frizzle in large skillet in butter, and brown on both sides:
5 eggs
1 c shrimp
1 c onions, chopped fine
¼ c water chestnuts, sliced thin
½ c mushrooms, sliced thin
2 T soy sauce

Serve with sauce made by simmering:
1 T soy sauce
1 t cornstarch
½ c bouillon
¼ t sugar
Yield: 6 servings

CHINESE VEGETABLE STEW

Brown in skillet in butter:
1 pound pork, sliced thin
Add and cook till golden brown:
2 T butter
1 medium onion, chopped
1 c bean sprouts
1 c thin-sliced celery
½ c mushrooms, thinly sliced
1 can bamboo shoots
Add and simmer 10 minutes:
2 c water
Add, stir in slowly, and cook till slightly thick:
1 T cornstarch
1 T water
Add to taste:
¼ c toasted almonds
2 T soy sauce
Serve over brown rice.
Yield: 6–8 servings

EGGS FOO YUNG

Stir and mix in moderate skillet for 1 minute.
½ pound mushrooms, sliced
2 T butter
Add and stir for about 5 minutes:
1 c sliced onions
1 c diced celery
Beat well:
4 eggs
¼ t salt
⅛ t pepper
Combine onion and egg mixtures and add:
¾ c bean sprouts
Melt in large skillet:
2 T butter
Drop egg mixture into skillet from a large spoon. Turn the cakes once. Serve with soy sauce or with pureed organically grown apricots.
Yield: 6 servings

CHINESE MEAT BALLS

Mix well in bowl:
 1 pound round steak, ground
 1 egg
 2 T whole grain flour
 1 t salt
 1½ T onion, chopped fine
Make into balls, roll in flour and frizzle in butter till a light brown. Add and simmer over low heat for a few minutes:
 ⅓ c chicken stock or water
  and powdered vegetable seasoning
 1 T butter
 4 slices pineapple, cubed
 3 green peppers cut in large pieces
Mix well and add to meat balls:
 1 T cornstarch
 2 t soy sauce
 ¼ c apple cider vinegar
 ⅛ c dark brown sugar

Heat until slightly thick and serve.
Yield: 4 servings

JELLIED DESSERT

Desserts are usually fresh fruits, but here is another dessert the Chinese occasionally eat.

Place in saucepan, bring to boil slowly and simmer 10 minutes:
 2 T agar-agar powder
 2½ c water
 2 T dark brown sugar
Add and simmer 5 minutes, stirring often:
 1½ t almond extract
 2 T dark brown sugar
 1¼ c sweetened condensed milk
Pour the mixture into a shallow, lightly greased cake pan, and cool; then place in fridge to set. To serve, cut almond-jelly into cubes and place in a large bowl with chunks of fresh fruit.

8

PLANT-PROTEIN MAIN DISHES

OVERVIEW

Let's talk about whole grains, nuts and seeds combined with legumes (beans, peas, peanuts) used as main dishes. (We'll consider breakfast grains and baked goods in the next chapter.) These plant proteins take the place of animal protein dishes for cancer patients during the crisis period, probably about three months until their cancer goes into remission. They can gradually eat small amounts of fish, and chicken from the health food store or from a farmer who raises chicken for his own family, without the commercial feed that contains hormones, additives and pesticides.

All through life, however, we should eat grains and beans in combination to furnish excellent protein to help keep us from getting cancer or any other degenerative disease. Let's remember that natural foods, well digested, are our first line of defense because they will help us have a healthy immune system so we can destroy precancerous cells and, if we need to, fight cancer itself.

We need to eat our grains whole—not refined—with the germ and bran left in. The germ of grains contains oils, proteins and vitamins, especially vitamin E. The cells of the grain are full of starch and protein. The bran is made up of several layers. The outside layer is mostly indigestible cellulose, but the four other layers have much less fiber and much more protein and vitamins, especially B1 and B3 (Ballentine, 1978).

We combine legumes—beans, peas and peanuts—with whole grains to make complete proteins. In addition to our usual reasons for eating legumes—they are excellent proteins—

they, along with lecithin, lower the incidence of heart attacks. Other foods do, too, especially whole grains, vegetables and garlic (Ballentine, 1978).

Beans and peas are "as near to being perfect vegetables as it is possible to find" (Seddon and Burrow, 1977). They have more starch for energy and more protein than other vegetables. Dried beans and peas, chickpeas and lentils have about 20 percent protein. They lack vitamin C but are a good source when sprouted. Mung beans are the ones most often eaten as sprouts. Beans and peas are high in iron and low in sodium.

Plant proteins can be made into everything from soup to desserts—casseroles, bean and nut loaves, and even sauces to go on the loaves. These combinations of plant proteins will make you forget you ever thought you had to have beef every day.

We have to know what we're doing when we combine grains and legumes to get high quality proteins. Let's borrow the wheels from Lesson 1 of *A Home Study Course in the New Nutrition* (Long, 1983). Figure 1 (p. 57) represents the protein value of whole grains, nuts and seeds. Every spoke in the circle represents one of the essential amino acids. We have to eat these all at one time to make a complete protein. You'll notice that one of the spokes is shorter than the rest. The short one limits the amount of protein we can get from the food to only as much as is in the one that's short. The small circle represents the protein value we get from those amino acids. The part of the spokes that sticks out beyond the circle can't be used as protein—it is used as energy or stored as fat. We can't afford to waste protein

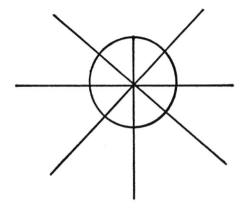

A. *whole grains,*
nuts, seeds

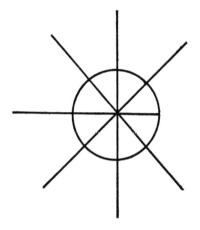

B. *legumes (beans,*
peas, peanuts)

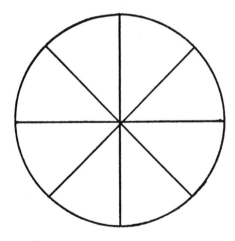

C. *eggs,*
dairy products,
animal proteins

Figure 1.
The amino acid pattern of proteins.

this way, so we combine grains with legumes, which are another good source of protein, but also incomplete. Legumes have one amino acid in short supply, but it's a different one from the one that's short in grains. When we eat grains and legumes together, we get complete protein because the amino acid that is short in grains is plentiful in legumes, and vice versa. Thus we get the protein represented in Circle 3—all eight amino acids in maximum amounts. This diagram also represents the protein value of eggs, dairy products and animal proteins, which are all complete proteins.

Obviously, Group C foods can be eaten by themselves because they're complete proteins, but they also have enough of all amino acids to complement plant proteins short in one amino acid.

Children need more protein in proportion to their size than adults, because children use protein for growth and repair; adults use it only for repair of tissue.

Combining foods this way gets to be second nature. Recently I looked at our plates at supper one night and all the protein we had was lentil soup—a legume. I had several choices of foods to complement the lentils, but the first thing that caught my eye when I went to the fridge was bran muffins, so we all ate some muffins. I could have served cheese, grains in other forms, eggs or a small amount of some other animal protein.

How much grain and legumes should we eat to get the right combination of amino acids? A rule of thumb is twice as much grains as legumes. So, if you're serving brown rice and pinto beans, eat ½ cup of brown rice with ¼ cup of beans if you're a little lady, or twice as much of each if you're a big man. The amino acids will be right.

What if you have lentil soup? It has lentils, a legume, but it has a lot of water in it. How do we know how much grain to eat? Let's just have two muffins and not worry about it. The main thing is to remember always to combine grains and legumes with each other or with some kind of animal protein.

GRAINS

Let's go over some of the most important grains used as main dishes all over the world.

AMARANTH

Amaranth is a rediscovered plant protein, now beginning to be distributed for food. It is high in protein, calcium and fiber. Usually we should eat a starch with it, such as arrowroot powder or Tapioca Starch Flour (not Minute Tapioca), soy, buckwheat, wholewheat or potato starch flour, or ground nuts or seeds. The suggested proportion is 75 percent amaranth with 25 percent of any of the starch flours. We'll have to remember not to combine it with wheat germ or bran as we often combine foods now. We can use wholewheat or ground nuts instead. If you want to try this new plant protein, write Illinois Amaranth Company, Dept C, Rural Route 2, Box 396-A, Mundelein, IL 60060 for information on ordering. You may order information about amaranth from Rodale Press, 33 E. Minor St., Emmaus, PA 18049.

BULGUR

Bulgur is parboiled whole cracked wheat. It still has the germ and bran; it's inexpensive, it cooks quickly and it's appetizing. One serving (about ¼ pound) has 11.2 grams of protein, 75 grams of carbohydrate, 1.5 grams of fat, and is very high in phosphorus and potassium.

Bulgur makes excellent pilaf, an Oriental dish made of grain cooked with some kind of animal protein and seasoned with spices. It's good served with meat and poultry, soups, hamburger, steamed pudding and in many other ways.

MILLET

Millet is new to almost everyone, but it's one of the best-tasting and most versatile grains. One-half cup of cooked millet has 10 grams of protein, but since it's incomplete, as are all the grains, we add dairy products or legumes. Millet looks like yellow rice when cooked. It has a different and delightful flavor. Millet is higher in protein than corn, barley, or sorghum. It is sometimes made into chapattis, a flat bread like tortillas (Seddon and Burrow, 1977).

BUCKWHEAT

Buckwheat is usually called groats. It is not related to wheat. It is about 11 percent protein, and just 2 percent fat. It is not made into bread or muffins, but it makes good pancakes. Added to wheat bread, it furnishes lysine, an amino acid in short supply in wheat. Buckwheat groats can be used as a rice substitute. Buckwheat flour makes super crepes or pancakes which can be frozen and reheated in the toaster oven. They're especially good made with yeast.

Kasha, another name for buckwheat, can be served with meat and vegetables and is especially good with yogurt. It's prepared the same as brown rice. We can buy it as groats and grind it fresh to flour in the blender; it's a soft grain and won't hurt the blades. Also, it grinds very fine. Toasted groats are dark and rich tasting (Ballentine, 1978).

BROWN RICE

Rice is the most popular grain; it's the main food of millions of people in the world. In many countries, rice is a good source of protein, but if we tried to live on the kind of rice most people eat here—white—we wouldn't do very well. We should eat brown rice with all the vitamins and minerals intact. White rice is polished and then dipped in nutrients which are supposed to replace some of those lost in the polishing. If we wash the rice, all those added nutrients can be lost. So read the directions on the label. Don't wash the rice unless the label tells you to, even brown rice. Almost all the fat and minerals are lost when brown rice is polished. The worst loss is vitamin B1, a deficiency of which causes beri-beri.

BARLEY

Pearl barley is not good; we use pot barley, which is whole grain. Pearl barley lacks most of the bran and germ. Barley makes excellent soup. Adding lentils makes a high protein dish.

Half of the barley in the world is fed to animals, and most of the rest is used for beer and whiskey. Wine was made from barley in 2800 B.C. Barley water is made by boiling barley in water and straining it. It is used for upset stomach and nervousness and for teething problems in children (Ballentine, 1978).

RYE

Rye is said to be good for dieters because it makes muscle, whereas wheat makes fat.

CORN

Corn is not as high in protein as wheat. Corn used to be the major food of many of the people in the South. This diet caused pellagra because the corn is deficient in niacin (vitamin B3). Niacin can be made from tryptophan, an amino acid, so if there is enough protein in the diet, niacin will not be deficient.

OATS

Oats taste better if roasted dry or with a little butter before adding water. They take about 45 minutes to an hour to cook this way.

PHYTIC ACID

Phytic acid in whole grains, beans and peas was once thought to combine with minerals, especially calcium, iron and zinc, and excrete them in the stool. But a report from research chemist Eugene R. Morris (*Houston Chronicle*, April, 1980) notes that human volunteers who ate whole wheat in normal amounts excreted less of the minerals. Morris reported to the annual meeting of the Federation of American Societies for Experimental Biology that the whole wheat actually helped the body absorb the minerals.

FREEZING GRAINS AND LEGUMES

It isn't any more trouble to cook large amounts of grains and beans than it is to cook small amounts. Freeze them in family-sized portions ready for your favorite recipe. Brown rice and barley take so long to cook (60 minutes), it's nice to have them in the freezer. Cracked wheat and bulgur take only about 15 minutes, so there's no need to cook them ahead.

NUTS AND SEEDS

Ounce for ounce, nuts and seeds supply almost twice the nutrient value of any other food. Nuts are very high protein. Peanuts, for example, are 26 percent protein. Next highest are cashews and walnuts. Also good are almonds, with 18 percent protein, low starch, 50 percent fat of the best kind, plus B vitamins and iron (Adams and Murray, 1973).

Sunflower seeds are the seeds highest in protein as well as in essential fatty acids and vitamin E. Close seconds are sesame and pumpkin seeds. Sesame seeds are high in calcium; most other seeds are high in phosphorus.

Buy raw nuts and seeds for best food value. Buy shelled nuts with the skin on, if they have skin, like almonds and peanuts. But if possible, buy nuts with the shells on and shell them yourself. If you just don't have time for that, at least buy them raw—not toasted, not "dry roasted," not salted. Don't forget, always roast peanuts; eat other nuts and seeds raw.

Roast peanuts at 300 degrees F for 30 minutes, stirring often toward the end of the time. There's more food value in other nuts and seeds if you eat them raw. If your family won't go for raw nuts, toast half and leave the other half raw. You'll get the better food value of the raw nuts and the better taste of the toasted nuts.

Chop and grind nuts just before eating them or using them in recipes. Otherwise, they're exposed to oxygen and can quickly become rancid.

In grinding seeds in a blender, it is best to start with about a cup. They grind better if not in too small amounts. But it's easy to grind a small amount in a seed and nut grinder. Thus you can prepare a few spoonfuls at a time—

they're fresh for youngsters and oldsters who might not be able to chew whole seeds.

Sprinkle seeds, especially pumpkin, sunflower and sesame seeds, on salads. White sesame seeds look the best.

It's amazing what toasted peanuts and Swiss cheese bits do for a plain green salad. Sunflower seeds soaked in cold water just to cover for about 15 minutes while you're preparing dinner pep up a salad so much that you'll never believe they're just plain little ol' sunflower seeds. Use them in cooked vegetables, too.

Since sesame seeds are high in calcium, use them often. But serve other nuts and seeds with vegetables or milk or with milk sauce for extra calcium.

Pulverized grains and seeds can be stirred into batters and bread doughs and sauces for higher protein content. Sprinkle ground nuts over vegetable casseroles. When seeds and grains are ground, they cook faster. Soybeans, lentils, split peas and others can be ground and used in soups, chowders, loaves and patties.

Several different grinders can do the job. Blenders are probably found in most kitchens. Then there are food processors, grinders, food mills and electric coffee grinders.

LEGUMES

Here's a quick list of beans: black, lima, great northern, kidney, navy, peabeans, pinto, red, pink and soy. Peas include black eyed, garbanzos, dry whole peas and dry split peas. Since legumes are not complete proteins, to get full protein value, combine legumes with nuts, seeds or whole grains or with animal proteins or dairy products.

When serving any beans, dress them up so your family will accept them enthusiastically. Lentils, peas, black beans and soybeans make good soups. Kidney beans and garbanzos (chickpeas) are good in salads or dips. Peabeans are seasoned with maple syrup and are called Boston baked beans.

Peanuts are probably the most popular legume, as well as one of the most healthful. But peanuts are very easily damaged by a mold called aspergillus flavus, which causes cancer. The actual poison is aflatoxin. It has caused cancer

in every species it has been tested on. Naturally, it can't be tested on humans. To assure our best chance of getting mold-free peanuts, it would probably be best to buy peanuts and peanut butter at health food stores. Besides avoiding aflatoxin, health food store peanut butter is made from toasted peanuts with a little salt added—none of the additives such as hydrogenated oil or sugar.

Peanut "spread" is made from a starchy mass flavored with chemicals that taste like peanuts, but which contains no peanuts! Buy from a recognized health food manufacturer and be sure you're getting only peanuts in your peanut butter.

Soybeans are 36 percent protein; other legumes are 20 to 24 percent and have almost twice as much carbohydrate. The oil is 51.5 percent linoleic acid, the one essential fatty acid the body can't manufacture and which we have to obtain from our food.

Soybeans can be bought as beans, of course, or as granules, powder or flour. These can all be used in main dishes and also to fortify many other recipes, making soy a good protein for your dollar (Walczak, 1977).

SPICES

To digest our vegetable proteins and make them taste good, too, Ballentine (1978) suggests using spices fried in clarified butter. The spices must not be heated to a high temperature or they may be so changed in structure that they are not healthful. The three most used spices in India are turmeric, cumin and coriander. These are mild and help us digest food and give a rich flavor to the dish. After they are heated in the butter, they are added to vegetables or beans. Turmeric is said to be healthful for the skin. Cumin is found in many Mexican dishes. It helps correct intestinal gas and is a remedy for colic or for headache caused by an upset stomach. More cumin is usually used than turmeric.

More coriander, however, is used than cumin. It is even used instead of cinnamon for apple pie. It is also used in medicines to mask an unpleasant taste. This spice also reduces gas in the intestinal tract.

Other seasonings—pepper, ginger, black mustard seeds, fenugreek—are useful. Besides tasting good and providing protein, beans cooked well help prevent arteriosclerosis and heart disease (Ballentine, 1978).

TIMETABLE FOR COOKING GRAINS

1 cup grains	water (cups)	time	yield (cups)
barley	3	1¼ h	3½
brown rice	2	1 h	3
buckwheat	2	15 m	2½
bulgur	2	15–20 m	2½
cracked wheat	2	25 m	2⅓
millet	3	45 m	3½
coarse cornmeal	4	25 m	3
wild rice	3	2 h	4
wholewheat berries	3	2 h	2⅔
wheat flakes	3	30 m	4
rolled oats	2	30 m	4

WHOLEGRAIN AND BEAN DISHES

COUSCOUS

The next time you see Paris, go to the left bank—to a short street named rue Xavier Privas. Almost every building on that street is a restaurant that specializes in couscous. It is an Algerian dish that should take the place of spaghetti at every church or Boy Scout supper in this land. Whereas spaghetti is a white flour junk food, couscous is made of whole grain millet. All they do to the grain is steam it and serve a huge mound of it with a deep pot of the best stew you ever ate. The stew can be all beef or any other meat or a combination. The seasonings bring out the best in the meat and in the chunks of tender vegetables.

Sear 1½ lbs. stew meat till brown and add water. Add salt and the following seasonings to taste:
    1 t oregano
    ½ t basil
    1 t tamari (soy sauce)
    1 bay leaf
Or
    salt and pepper to taste

Or
    try East Indian seasonings:
After searing the meat, remove it from the pan. On medium heat, stir in one at a time and heat till slightly brown:
    1 t turmeric
    2 t cumin
    3 t ground coriander
Don't burn. Return the meat to the pan and add water. Simmer the meat till almost tender and test for seasonings. Add if needed:
    salt and pepper

Steam in a deep pan:
    2 c millet (bulgur can also be used)
    6 c water
    sea salt to taste
Don't stir while cooking. This takes about 45 minutes.

Add to stew meat and simmer until tender one or more of the following vegetables:
    1 large carrot sliced thin
    1 rib celery, sliced thin
    1 green pepper seeded and cubed
    1 c peas (fresh if possible)
    1 c green beans (1" pieces)
    1 c shredded red cabbage
    1 c broccoli flowerets
Add and cook five minutes longer:
    ½ c button mushrooms
    1 c cooked dried chickpeas

Serve the millet in soup plates. Each person helps himself to stew. The beauty of this meal is that it can be made without meat. Also, any vegetable not available can be omitted and others substituted. Any dried beans can be cooked, seasoned well and served with the millet, which makes a complete protein.
Yield: 6–8 servings

WHOLEGRAIN SOUFFLE

Preheat oven to 350 F. Mix and beat lightly:
    3 egg yolks
    1¾ c cooked millet or other whole grain
    ½ t sea salt
    ⅔ c grated sharp cheese
    ⅔ c milk

Beat until stiff and fold into millet mixture:
  3 egg whites
Pour into a 1½ quart casserole. Set dish in a pan of hot water and bake about 20 minutes or until set.
Yield: 6 servings

To reheat, wrap soufflé in foil and place in steamer; steam at low temperature to avoid excess steam and water, which collects in the top pan.

Sprinkle fresh grated cheese on top before serving.

Or: Wrap soufflé slices in foil, heat at 300 F in toaster-oven about 20 minutes.

WHOLEGRAIN STEW

Cook covered for 45 minutes:
  1 c whole millet or other grain
  1 t tamari (soy sauce)
  3 c boiling water
Steam in steamer one or more vegetables, for a total of two cups:
  onion
  parsley
  cabbage
  green peppers
  winter squash, peeled and cubed
Add vegetables to cooked grain with:
  1–2 T butter
  1 c shredded sharp cheese
  salt and pepper to taste
Yield: 6 servings

CHEESY GRAIN CASSEROLE

Cook covered for 45 minutes (or see Timetable for Cooking Grains, p. 61)
  3 c boiling water
  1 c millet or other grain
Add to cooked millet:
  3 well-beaten eggs
  1½ c milk
  1 c grated sharp cheese
  1 t vegetable salt
Pour into a shallow baking dish, bake at 350 F till set—about 45 minutes.
Yield: 6 servings

Or: Everything the same except use corn grits (1 cup) cooked in 4 c boiling water for 25 minutes.

FRIZZLED MILLET

Use "prepared ahead" millet that you packed in a square refrigerator dish. Slice the millet and frizzle in butter in a moderate skillet. If you like, sprinkle the sesame seeds in the skillet and cook the millet slices on top.
Yield: 2–4 servings

NO-MEAT LOAF

Some of my nutrition students made this loaf and served it to husband and children, who all thought it was meat loaf. This might be an easy way to Switchover to good nutrition.

Preheat oven to 350 F.
Blend in blender till finely ground, then place in bowl:
  1 c walnuts or pecans
Add:
  1 c wheat germ
  1 c grated mild cheddar cheese
Blend in blender:
  ¾ c milk or tomato juice
  3 eggs
  1 large onion
  1 t thyme
  ¼ t marjoram
  ½ t sea salt
Pour blender mix over bowl mix. Stir well. Turn into an oiled loaf pan 9×5×3". Bake 45 minutes.
Yield: 6–8 servings

FLUFFY BROWN RICE

Long grain brown rice is best for rice dinner dishes, plain boiled rice and pilaf. Short and medium grain are best for puddings and stuffings because they're sticky.

When you cook brown rice, add one tablespoon of butter to prevent its boiling over. As rice cooks, little passageways form through which steam escapes. The rice cooks dry and fluffy. But if you stir the rice, the passageways are closed up, and the steam can't escape. Then the rice will be sticky.

Measure 1 c raw rice into a large saucepan; it will triple in volume. Add 2 c boiling water, and return to boil. Cover and cook on very low heat for 45 minutes. Do not salt; do not stir. Remove from heat and let stand 10 minutes.
Variation: Stir raw rice in a medium hot skillet till toasted. Then cook as above. This rice has a nutty flavor.
Or: Add bits of vegetables, bean sprouts, and pine nuts or toasted peanuts.
Or: Sauté in butter, in separate pan, one medium onion, chopped, and 2 to 4 T chopped parsley. Cook the raw rice till half done, sprinkle sauteed vegetables on top of rice with ½ c raisins or other dried fruit and chopped nuts. Do not stir. Finish cooking and stir lightly.
Yield: Four to six servings.

GRAINS, VEGETABLES AND CHEESE

Preheat oven to 350 F. Steam for 5 minutes:
    2 large carrots, sliced thin
    1 small onion, sliced
Combine the following and add to carrots:
    2 eggs, lightly beaten
    1 pound cottage cheese
    1 c cooked grain
    ½ t sea salt
    ½ t marjoram
Turn into buttered casserole. Sprinkle with:
    ½ c grated cheese
    paprika
    ½ c wheat germ
Bake 45 minutes. For two people, use two small loaf pans; eat one, freeze one.
Yield: 6 servings

BROWN RICE AND FRUIT

Sauté:
    ¼ c chopped onion in ½ stick butter
Add and stir for a few minutes:
    1 c raw brown rice or cracked wheat
Add and simmer rice 45 minutes, cracked wheat 15 minutes (do not stir):
    2 c chicken stock or vegetable stock
Add, fluff and serve:
    ½ c slivered almonds sautéed in butter
    1 c lightly steamed chopped dried apricots or fresh chopped apple

Toast the almonds in the toaster-oven if you wish.
Yield: 4–6 servings

MORE EASY GRAIN DISHES

1. Paella: Steam onion and green pepper in a little butter. Add pieces of steamed chicken, soy bean bits, beef, tuna, leftover shrimp or other animal or vegetable foods of your choice. Serve over brown rice.

2. Add to steamed grains shortly before serving:
    ½ c cooked corn or vegetable
    4 scallions, chopped
    ¾ c roasted peanuts

3. Toast whole grain for 5 minutes in a skillet with:
    2 T butter, then stir in:
    2 T chopped onion
    1 T parsley
    grated rind of ½ lemon
    2 T mixed herbs (tarragon, thyme, marjoram and/or basil)
Add water and finish cooking (about 40 minutes if you're using brown rice).

4. To cooked rice, millet, or cracked wheat, add:
    chopped omelet made of 2 eggs
    cooked peas or carrots
    onion and parsley, simmer in 1 T butter
    1 T tamari soy sauce

5. To cooked grains, add:
    onion and garlic simmered in 1 T butter
    ¼ t ground cumin
    ½ t chili powder
    ¼ c peanuts, toasted
    Leftover meat or fish or both

6. To cooked millet or other grain, add in layers:
    cooked stew meat
    and raisins combined

7. To cooked whole grains, add:
    seedless raisins
    chopped walnuts
    ground nutmeg
    chopped dried apricots
    chicken stock

8. To cooked cracked wheat, add:
   1 c sliced mushrooms
   ½ c grated cheddar cheese
   chicken or vegetable stock to taste

9. To cooked grain, add:
   1 stalk celery, chopped
   ⅓ c chopped cashews
   ⅓ c seedless raisins
Serve hot or cold.
Yield from 2 c steamed grains: 3–4 servings

Leftover grains can be kept a day or two in the fridge. To warm up, frizzle in a pan with butter, stirring constantly, put the top on the pan and turn the burner off. In a few minutes, the grains will be moist and fresh.

WHEAT GERM AS AN "ADDITIVE"

Wheat germ is one of the best "additives" we have. Here are some suggestions to add protein, vitamins and minerals to your food preparation.

1. Add to any baked goods. Substitute wheat germ for one-fourth of the flour. The bread will be slightly heavier because it will not rise as much whether made with yeast or baking powder.

2. Add wheat germ to the granola you buy.

3. Wheat germ is always ready to coat frizzled foods or foods to be broiled or baked.

4. Sprinkle wheat germ on top of casseroles, with cheese or without. Add paprika for taste and color.

5. Make your own shake-on coating with seasoned wheat germ. Add sea salt to taste, herbs or powdered vegetable seasoning from the health food store or other favorite spices or seasonings.

6. Sprinkle wheat germ on yogurt. Flavor with your own fresh, raw, ripe fruit.

CREPES

Many grains may be used to make crepes. After they're made, they can be easily frozen.

Cool the crepes and stack them, then put the whole stack in a plastic bag. They will usually separate easily if you help them along by twisting a knife blade between them while they're still frozen hard. It's safer to put waxed paper or plastic wrap between them. Save the sheets in the freezer, and the next time you make crepes (or pancakes) use the same sheets in between. Add fillings when defrosted and ready to serve. To speed up the defrosting, warm them in a toaster-oven. They're good for breakfast just warmed with butter.

WHOLEGRAIN CREPES

Blend all ingredients together and whirl in blender on low:
   1 c buttermilk, milk or yogurt.
   1 c water
   1¼ c wholewheat flour
   ½ c fine cornmeal
   1 t grated orange peel
   5 eggs
   ½ t salt
   2 T soft butter
   1 T honey (optional)
Cook in skillet or crepe pan.

Or: Instead of wholewheat flour and corn meal, use 1¾ c wholewheat flour or part buckwheat.
Yield: up to 40 small crepes

FILLINGS FOR CREPES

1. Mashed, seasoned beans with grated cheese.
2. Curried creamed chicken or fish.
3. Pureed, seasoned cooked vegetables.
4. Ricotta or cottage cheese flavored with fruit.
5. Applesauce or home-frozen or fresh peaches with yogurt.
6. Yogurt, cottage cheese, crushed strawberries, with 1–2 t brown sugar.

Roll enough crepes (except sweet crepes) for a baking dish and cover with grated cheese or cheese sauce browned a minute under the broiler. The whole pan full can be prepared in advance then reheated in a moderate oven covered tightly with foil.

Or: Stack 6 to 8 crepes with filling between. Cut into slices like pie. This is easy and fast, and the stacks look pretty.

Or: Use tortillas instead of crepes; spread each with homemade chili (p. 44) sprinkled with grated, natural cheese. Serve with vegetable salad.
Yield: 6–8 servings

HYPRO "SAUSAGE" PATTIES

Mix together, chill and form into 8 medium patties:
    2 c cooked bulgur and soy grits, mixed
    1 egg
    ¼ c wholewheat flour
    ¾ t black pepper
    1 T crushed basil leaves
    ¾ t sage
    ¾ t poultry seasoning
    sea salt to taste
Roll in wholewheat flour, frizzle in butter in skillet.

Or: Form into cocktail-size balls and serve with sweet-sour sauce. Add ¾ c grated cheddar cheese (optional).
Yield: 4–6 servings

GRAIN OR BEAN BURGERS

Preheat oven to 350 F. Use any beans, leftover grains or both combined. In blender:
    2 c cooked beans or grains
      or a combination of both
    1 small onion, finely chopped
    2 eggs
    1 T vegetable broth seasoning
    1 T tamari (soy sauce)
    1 c wheat germ
    ½ c ground sunflower seeds
Blend till smooth, spoon small amounts onto a lightly oiled baking sheet. Bake about 20 minutes.

Or: Add wheat germ or bread crumbs till mixture is consistency to pat into burgers. Roll in or sprinkle with sesame seeds. Frizzle in butter.

Or: Add ¼ c cottage cheese or Swiss cheese.

Or: Add nuts and/or raisins or other dried fruit.

Or: Serve with pureed home-frozen or fresh peaches or other fruit.
Yield: 6–8 servings

TIMETABLE FOR COOKING BEANS

1 cup beans	water (cups)	time	yield (cups)
black eyed peas	3	1 h	2
garbanzos	4	3 h	2
Great Northern	3½	2 h	2
kidney beans	3	1½ h	2
lima beans	2	1½ h	1¼
baby limas	2	1½ h	1¾
pinto beans	3	2½ h	2
red beans	3	3 h	2
navy beans	2	1½ h	2
soybeans	3	3 h	2
soy grits	4	15 m	2
lentils	3	1 h	2¼
split peas	3	1 h	2¼

DRIED BEANS

Prepare beans easily:
1. Pick over and wash in cold water.
2. Soak overnight in water which is three times the volume of beans. (Don't soak lentils and split peas.) For a quick method without soaking overnight, bring beans and water to a boil, cook two minutes, remove from heat, cover and let soak two hours.
3. After soaking overnight or two hours, bring beans and water to a boil, reduce heat to very low, cover and simmer gently about two hours or till tender. Fast cooking causes the beans to break. Split peas and lentils will be done in about 45 minutes.
4. Add salt when beans are almost tender. Salt added early makes beans tough. Never add baking soda.

GASLESS BEANS

Soak beans in water overnight. Pour off water. Add more water and bring to a simmer; pour off second water. Add more water and finish cooking. This method destroys more nutrients, but you can make up for that by adding 1 teaspoon of brewer's yeast for every ½ c of dried beans. I don't like the taste of yeast, but I can't taste it in beans cooked this way.

SOYBEANS

Soybeans are very healthful, but they need a lot of seasoning to taste good. Freeze them overnight in the kettle you'll cook them in. Cook by methods given. Serve in the following sauce.

Steam together:
  1 T butter
  1 small chopped onion
  1 chopped green pepper
Add and simmer, then add to beans:
  ½ c shredded jack, Swiss, or cheddar cheese
  ½ to 1 t chili powder
  ½ c tomato sauce
Yield: about 1 cup

TOFU PATTIES

Tofu is made from soybeans. Buy it at health food stores.

Steam until slightly tender:
  1 onion, chopped
  1 carrot, grated
  1 rib celery, chopped
Combine with:
  1 pound tofu, mashed
  2 T wheat germ
  ½ t salt
  2 T wholewheat flour
  1 t caraway seeds
Form into small patties or drop from spoon onto buttered cookie sheet. Bake at 350 F about 10 minutes each side, or roll in wheat germ and sauté in buttered skillet till brown.
Yield: 4 servings

BEANY MEXICAN ENCHILADAS

Set oven at 350 F. Steam for about 30 minutes until onions are tender:
  1 c cooked dry lima or red beans
  1 onion, chopped
  1 green pepper, chopped
  2 large or 6 small fresh-frozen tomatoes

1 T chili powder
1 t cumin powder or 2 t cumin seeds
salt to taste
½ c red wine
In buttered baking dish, place layers of:
  tortillas
  bean sauce
  a mixture of:
    3 T grated light cheddar cheese
    ½ c grated jack cheese
    ½ c yogurt
End with tortillas topped with cheese mixture.
Bake 15–20 minutes.
Yield: 6 servings

GARBANZO LOAF OR PATTIES

There's something really special about the flavor of garbanzo beans, also called chickpeas. Try them in this super loaf:

Preheat oven to 350 F. Mash by hand or processor (steel blade) and turn into large bowl:
  3 c cooked dried chickpeas or garbanzos
Add remaining ingredients:
  1 c chopped celery
  1 c wholewheat bread crumbs
    or part wheat germ
  1 c ground nuts (walnuts, almonds, pecans)
  2 T chopped parsley
  sea salt to taste
  1 T soy sauce
  2 T soy flour
  1 t sage
  2 T melted butter
  2 eggs, lightly beaten
  pinch black pepper
Turn into a buttered 9×5×3″ loaf pan and bake 30 minutes or until set.

Or: Drop by spoonfuls on a buttered skillet, turn once and serve.

Or: Substitute 1 c cooked millet or other whole grain for the bread crumbs and/or wheat germ.

Or: Use any kind of beans, grains or a combination of beans and grains.
Yield: 8–10 servings

This recipe can be as varied as our tastes. Choose different seasonings, spices, herbs, powdered vegetable seasonings from the health food store, sprouts, nuts ground or chopped and other special seasonings that your family prefers. Other suggestions are in More Easy Grain Dishes in this chapter, and in Salad Fixings, p. 95. We are limited only by our imaginations. You will probably become famous for your delightful "new" recipes. Actually, they are as old as man!

EAST INDIAN SPICED BEANS

Here's an East Indian bean recipe that's spicy and not gaseous. Ballentine (1978) gave permission for me to use this recipe. See References, p. 147.

Pick over 2 c of your favorite variety of beans—mung, soy, pintos, red, white or other. These may not be what East Indians would eat, but they all taste good. Wash beans in lukewarm water. Soak overnight for better digestibility.

Cook 15 minutes or more in a pressure cooker or till done in ordinary pan. While beans are cooking, put 3 T clarified butter in an iron skillet on medium heat.

Add 1 t turmeric, 2 t cumin, and 3 t ground coriander and stir until brown—don't burn. You can add mustard seed or grated ginger root if you wish. Add 1 large sliced onion and 1 c sliced mushrooms (both optional) and stir until brown. Add green pepper and tomatoes if you wish. The darker brown the vegetables and spices are, the more flavor the beans will have. Again, don't let them burn.

Add the spices to the beans, adding 1½ t salt, and water if needed. Cook the mixture 5 minutes or till the beans are soft and the mixture soupy.

In India, only about ½ c or less is eaten with a meal. This is used as a sauce for grains or as a dip for bread.
Yield: 8 half-cup servings

MEXICAN BEAN TREAT

Preheat oven to 450 F. Mix well and pour into a lightly greased 9 × 12″ baking pan:

2 c juicy heated beans (red or pinto)
1 t chili powder (or to taste)
2 t cumin seed or 1 t cumin powder
½ t sea salt (or to taste)
Mix in a large bowl:
1 c cornmeal
1 t baking soda
½ t salt
Mix well, then add to cornmeal mixture and stir till smooth:
2 c buttermilk
1 egg
2 T soft butter
Pour the batter over the beans and bake on the top rack of your oven until bread is golden brown and the bread leaves the sides of the pan; about 30 minutes.

This recipe serves six people well. It is easy to freeze. Cut into pieces that fit your toaster oven, wrap in foil (dull side of foil next to food), freeze and reheat. Double the recipe if you wish.

NUTS, SEEDS, SPROUTS

NUT AND SEED BUTTERS

Roast shelled peanuts in the oven just below 200 degrees F for about two hours. Grind in a blender till powdery. Gradually add butter, a teaspoonful at a time, until it's the consistency you like. Add a little salt and honey if you like. Add a few whole nuts and blend until lightly chopped if you like chunky peanut butter.

Any other nut or seed butters are just as easy to make. Use raw nuts other than peanuts; always toast peanuts. Try sesame seeds to make tahini, or any one of these: cashews, almonds, sunflower seeds, pecans or walnuts.

All nuts and seeds should be kept in the fridge or freezer. You can eat them right out of the freezer—they're hard and chewy, but good.

COCONUT

Coconut should be used more than it is. If you've forgotten the delicious taste of coconut, try it again—fresh. Pierce the eyes with an ice pick, drain milk, and drink it while frosty. Heat the coconut in a 400 F oven for 15 minutes. Put it in a plastic bag and hit it with a hammer (on the driveway) to break it in pieces. Use a sharp knife or a potato peeler to cut off the brown skin. Grate in a processor (steel blade or grater disc) and freeze. Add to cookie or muffin recipes.

SPROUTS

Sprouts are high-protein green foods. Buy seeds to sprout at your health food store. You'll find alfalfa seeds are about the easiest, but mung beans are easy, too. Both are useful in many ways. Navy beans, soy and kidney beans, as well as wheat and most other grains, make good sprouts.

To sprout seeds, soak about 1 T of seeds in a jar in the cupboard overnight. The jar should have either a piece of cheesecloth over the top held by a rubber band, or an old piece of nylon stocking. Health food stores have a special screen top that fits a standard size jar. The next day pour off the water and turn the jar upside down in a bowl at a slight tilt so it will drain well.

Rinse the sprouts at least twice a day and always put them back in the cupboard to drain. After 3 to 5 days, alfalfa seeds will have sprouted and will be 1 to 1½ inches long. Then bring them out in the light so the little leaves will turn a bright green.

These sprouts are especially good on a peanut butter sandwich on homemade wholewheat bread. They can also be put in tossed salads.

Mung beans are the steamed sprouts you eat in Chinese restaurants. Rye and wheat seed sprouts are dried and used to sweeten bread. Let sprouts get 1 inch long; dry them in a very slow oven at 150 degrees F for about an hour. Watch closely; don't let them burn. Store in covered jar in fridge.

Soybean sprouts should be boiled for exactly two minutes before storing since they contain an enzyme that destroys vitamin C in storage (Adams and Murray, 1973).

HOW TO USE SPROUTS

Sprouts are easy to use. You'll probably put them in everything (nearly), but for specific suggestions, try these:

1. Alfalfa, lentil or radish sprouts in salad with chopped carrots and Romaine leaves.
2. Alfalfa, lentil or mung bean sprouts in scrambled eggs.
2. Alfalfa or lentil sprouts in cucumber salad.
4. Salad greens and sprouted chickpeas tossed with lemon juice and sesame seeds.

SWEET AND SOUR SPROUTS

Let water come to a boil in bottom pan of steamer, then steam in top pan for one minute:
  2 c mung bean sprouts
sprinkled with:
  1 T sugar
  ½ t salt
Combine and pour over sprouts:
  1 T dark brown sugar
  2 T olive oil
  2 T apple cider vinegar
  dash black pepper
Store in fridge overnight. The sprouts will keep about a week in the fridge.
Yield: 2–4 servings

DRIED SPROUTS

Wheat, rye, soy, sesame and alfalfa sprouts all dry well. Spread sprouts on a cookie sheet and leave in a warm room or in a slightly heated oven (about 150 F) until they are dry. Grind the dried sprouts in a blender and store in a tightly covered jar. This powder can be used to enrich yogurt, baked goods, baby foods, nut butters and desserts. The powder keeps well.

SPROUTS FOR SWEETS

Dry soybean, garbanzo or pea sprouts to use as snacks or to mix with any cookie dough to enrich the vitamin and mineral content.

Place sprouts in a single layer in a baking pan. Bake at 350 F about ½ hour until sprouts are golden brown. You may like them sprinkled with brewer's yeast or a little powdered vegetable seasoning.

SPROUTED WHEAT BREAD

Sprouts for bread should be allowed to grow no longer than the seed itself. If too big, they contain so much water that the bread might be soggy.

Mix in a large bowl:
  1 c lukewarm water
  2 T dry yeast
Add:
  2 c lukewarm water
  1 T salt
  ¼ c honey or dark brown sugar
  3 T soft butter
Allow the yeast to bubble. Stir in:
  3½ c wholewheat flour
Beat well, cover and let rise until double. Add and knead well:
  1 c ground wheat sprouts
  1 c wheat sprouts, whole
  2 c wholewheat flour
Place in clean buttered bowl, cover and let rise in warm place till double. Punch down, knead and add more flour if necessary. Form into 2 loaves and place in buttered 7 × 3 × 2″ pans. Set oven at 350 F. Allow to rise, then bake for 40 to 60 minutes. Remove from pans and cool on wire rack.
Yield: 2 small loaves

SPROUT SPREAD

Chop coarsely and mix well in blender:
  1 c alfalfa or other sprouts (good choices are alfalfa, garbanzo and mung beans)
  2 to 3 T mixed cottage cheese and yogurt
  1 small onion
  1 T lemon juice
  ½ t salt or to taste
Spread on crackers, top with chopped eggs, olives, meats or seafood.
Yield: about 1¼ cups

SPROUTS FOR BREAKFAST

Prepare 1 c dried wheat, rye or alfalfa sprouts or a mixture. Mix well with 1 c oatmeal and cook according to the directions for the oatmeal.
Yield: 4 servings

SPROUT SANDWICH SPREAD

Mix well:
  ¼ c chopped onion
  ½ c chopped celery
  Sesame seed dressing (p. 96) to taste
  ½ c any sprouts (mung bean, lentil, alfalfa or a mixture)
Or: Add mashed or sliced avocado.
Yield: Enough for 2 sandwiches

9

BREAD AND BREAKFAST GRAINS

IN GENERAL

For breakfast and bread making, we have lots of choices of whole grain cereals from the health food store.

Whole grains are "foods of incomparable perfection" says Josef Issels, cancer specialist in Germany (Issels, 1975). But grains that have been refined have so little food value they should not take up space in our stomachs.

About 200 years ago, almost all flour was whole grain. Then when it was discovered how to remove the bran and germ and make white flour, it became a status symbol to eat white bread, and only the rich could afford it. Now, wholewheat bread is so perishable and white bread is so cheap that the roles are reversed. Often, wholewheat bread is so expensive that only the wealthy can afford it, and white bread is cheap enough for anyone to buy (Hunter, 1971).

We hear a lot about unbleached flour, but we don't want to buy that any more than white. First of all, with 70, 80 or 90 percent extraction, which means that 70 to 90 percent of the total quantity of the wheat is left in the flour, we lose the best 10 to 30 percent, which is the bran and germ. One hundred percent extraction is whole wheat.

Flour is bleached with chlorine dioxide which either destroys all the vitamin E left in the flour after it is milled, or forms a toxic product with methionine, an amino acid. This flour has been called a substance as nearly non-nutritious as it is possible to find (Hunter, 1971).

It's not just what's taken out of white flour that makes it so bad—sometimes it's what's put in. There are nearly 60 chemicals that may be used in bread without being stated on the label. A substitute for butter is used which needs no refrigeration; it does not spoil, and only one ounce flavors 60 pounds of dough. Then there's nitric acid, which colors some breads to make them look as if eggs were used.

Additives puff up bread and make the volume larger. We pay for air. Flour now is only 50 percent of the average loaf; 25 percent of the average cake. Wheat and rye bread average about 50 percent carbohydrate. Rye bread is more filling than wheat, so you may eat less (Seddon and Burrow, 1977). But be sure to make it yourself.

The baking industry uses more sugar than any other user. Other harmful additives are the sodium salt of propionic acid—harmful because of its extra sodium content. It doesn't help to use the calcium salt of propionic acid, because the enzyme that helps the body assimilate the calcium in the bread is destroyed.

So much information has been published about the poor food value of white flour that probably everybody knows about that. But many people still think wholewheat flour and bread from the supermarket are good.

Omohundro (1979) published an eye-opening report on what's wrong with commercial wholewheat. First, if the label says "wheat flour," that's white flour. Next, even if you find a label that says "100 percent whole wheat," the flour gets 410 times the pesticide dosage of white flour because vermin like the wholewheat flour best.

Then, the mill automatically separates bran, germ and white flour. To make it "whole" again, the three parts are put back together. But the molecules of all three parts have been changed by the pressure and heat of the rolling mill.

Have you found a label that says "100 percent stone ground wholewheat flour"? It should be good, but "Don't bet on it" says Omohundro. That researcher couldn't find any bread on the market which is made from organically grown, non-sprayed, non-fungicide wheat.

Another report in the *Journal of Applied Nutrition* by Beatrice Trum Hunter (1980) revealed the use of fumigants and solvents in food processing. Wheat and wheat flour are fumigated with ethylene oxide (EO), which causes severe nutrient destruction. Almost all the B vitamins are lost, plus histadine and methionine—amino acids. Methyl bromide is used to fumigate flour, stored grains and other foods. Residues of as much as 400 ppm of EO are found in dried eggs and spices; 125 ppm in bread, biscuit, cake, cookie and pie mixes, cereal flour, cracked rice, barley flour, oats, rice, macaroni and noodle products and soy flour.

FORTIFYING GRAINS

We should always fortify whole grain products we make because grains are low in the amino acid lysine. It's easy—just add wheat germ, soy powder or non-instant powdered milk to the bread or cereal. Add about two tablespoons of whichever you choose to one cup of grain. There is more total protein in soy flour, but there are more essential amino acids in non-instant powdered skim milk. Non-instant skim milk has much more food value than instant because instant is processed at a high temperature which destroys more nutrients.

Soy powder should be used rather than soy flour. Soy flour, the same as all other legumes, has a substance in it that destroys a digestive enzyme. That substance has been removed in the powder. In addition to fortifying cereals, a teaspoon of soy powder can be used to fortify a milk drink.

Never buy white flour, white rice or white crackers. You get far less for your money from these so-called foods than from any other form of grain or cereal (Walczak, 1977).

Avoid rye bread unless you make it. Commercial rye is just about equal to commercial white bread. In fact, we never use any cereal or grain product from the supermarket because they've been so processed that much of the food value is destroyed. When any grain is ground, it quickly begins to deteriorate and it becomes rancid, even if kept in the fridge. It keeps well if frozen (Ballentine, 1978).

We use only wholegrain flour for bread. It makes rather heavy bread, but it has a delicious flavor. Bread flour is made from hard wheat and has gluten in it. This bread will rise with yeast. Yeast is a microorganism that grows when it lives in warm liquids. As it grows, it produces carbon dioxide, which makes the dough rise. Yeast can be stored in a sealed plastic bag in the fridge for up to two weeks and in the freezer for up to one year.

To add yeast to bread, dissolve 1 teaspoon of sugar in a little lukewarm water, then add the yeast. It will foam up in five or ten minutes. The yeast will work without the sugar, but it will not foam up. Dried yeast will keep for up to six months if stored in an airtight container in a cool, dry place. One tablespoon of dried yeast equals one fresh yeast cake.

Salt is usually used at the rate of ½ teaspoon to every cup of flour. Too much salt slows down the growth of the yeast. The liquid used can be water or milk, or a combination of both. The liquid should be tepid. If too hot, it will kill the yeast. Add it all at one time. If too sticky, add more flour.

Fat, eggs and molasses or honey may be added. Butter improves the flavor of bread and helps it stay fresh longer. Eggs give bread a rich flavor.

How to store bread? Risen dough may be put in a greased bowl, covered with greased plastic and kept about two days before being cooked. It also may be frozen, but it is better to use 50 percent more yeast than the recipe calls for. Put the dough in a greased plastic bag, insert a straw, and suck out the air before sealing the bag. This way, unrisen dough may be frozen for one to two months; risen dough for one month. Baked yeast bread keeps in the freezer at 0 degrees F for six to eight months; baked quick bread two to three months. The bread must be completely cool before being wrapped in foil or sealed in a plastic bag.

QUICK BREADS

Yeast bread is not the only kind of bread we make. Quick breads are delicious—light, fluffy wheat germ muffins, banana and other fruit breads, rich biscuits, crispy crackers, cheese straws, corn dodgers or muffins all satisfy our need for natural whole grains.

Take an hour or two off once in a while and bake ahead. The freezer will keep these breads as fresh as the day you baked them, and you can warm up a different kind every day in the toaster oven.

The best kind of flour for quick breads and cakes is pastry flour. It is made from soft wheat, and it won't rise with yeast because soft wheat contains little or no gluten. To make the breads light, we need to stir the batter just enough to make the flour disappear and then pop it in a pre-heated oven as quickly as possible. Once you have the ingredients out of the freezer, you can turn out six recipes almost as easily as one. You don't have to wash the bowls and utensils in between, and it doesn't take any longer to clean up the kitchen!

Quick breads are made with one of the three kinds of baking powder:
1. Tartaric acid (from grapes) begins action at room temperature as soon as liquid is added.
2. Phosphate acts slowly and requires heat.
3. Double acting: acts the most slowly and releases one-third of its rising ability with liquid and ⅔ with heat.

We should avoid aluminum compounds.

You can make your own baking powder. Use two cups each of arrowroot flour and cream of tartar, and one cup of potassium bicarbonate from the drug store. Sift together, store in a tightly closed jar, and use the same as commercial powder. If you buy baking powder, buy it at the health food store.

I told a friend about making her own bread, and she said she just couldn't. Then I suggested she make bran muffins. The next time I saw her, she said she had been serving bran muffins to all her guests, and they loved them. They are easy to make.

You're probably thinking, "I'll never have time for all of this." But you will. On this new natural food diet, you'll have so much energy you'll have to move around. You might as well move into the kitchen and turn out batches of good bakery products in no time at all. However, I suggest hiring a cook one day (or half day) a month. She could make enough baked goods to last your family a month. A cook could work for 20 different families and everyone profits!

BREAKFAST GRAINS

We don't eat cereals in packages or boxes from the supermarket. The grains are heated to very high temperatures—up to 392 degrees F—and some amino acids and B vitamins are lost. By the time many of the cereals are processed, the carbohydrate content ranges from 70 to 88 percent. Many contain more sugar than grain (Hunter, 1971). Sweetened cereals are among the worst foods, and the price is much higher than for unsweetened cereals. Most are preserved with BHA and BHT and have added color. Granola is good if unsweetened, but it may be hard to find. Make your own and sweeten it with raisins. Adding fresh coconut just before eating it is really a treat.

Many manufacturers emphasize the protein content of dry cereals, probably because people will pay more for high-protein cereals. But an average cooked cereal has twice as much protein as an average ready-to-eat cereal.

Frosted rice cereal used to have so much iron added that the flakes could be moved around with magnets. The manufacturers removed some of the iron, and now they say the flakes can't be moved with magnets unless they are "very, very strong magnets" (McGovern Committee Report, V, page 30).

As breakfast cereals, there are enough different grains available that you won't have to eat the same one twice in ten days. Try these on your family.

WHEAT: whole berries, wheat flakes, or cracked wheat
BULGUR: a partially cooked wheat
RYE: flakes, grind whole rye in blender to make flour
BUCKWHEAT: a soft grain that can be ground in your own blender without damaging the blades. Make buckwheat pancakes and crepes
OATS: a cereal with 16 percent protein. The

best grain protein, with a lot of food value for your dollar because of its excellent vitamin and mineral content. Don't buy refined or quick oats. Do get the long cooking kind. Steel cut are best because they're not heated to a high temperature in the manufacture (Davis, 1947). Oatmeal is good for people with diabetes or digestive problems such as colitis. It's low in sodium. Grind your own oat flour in the blender.

CORN: usually used as meal—stone ground

WHEAT GERM: vacuum packed or nitrogen packed to insure freshness. Enriches other cereals with extra protein. Very high in lysine (whole grains are low in this nutrient).

POPCORN: for a breakfast the kids can't resist, pop the corn in a hot air popper to avoid using oil, break it up in the blender and serve with whole milk and raisins.

MILLET: although excellent as a meat substitute, millet is also good as a breakfast cereal with chopped dates or date sugar and milk.

SOY: not a grain, but a legume. It fortifies well all the above grains. Go slowly; people may not like the taste of soy at first.

Most people eat cereals with milk, which adds the missing amino acid, lysine, if the milk is not pasteurized at too high a temperature. You may cook the grains in milk and add butter, wheat germ, nuts and fruit. A good habit to get into is to add from 1 teaspoon to 1 tablespoon of non-instant powdered milk to every serving of whole grains after they're cooked.

All these whole grains are excellent complex carbohydrates. They're healthful because they're starches rather than sugars. Several studies show that blood fats and arteriosclerosis are lowered when starches are eaten, if the starches are complex carbohydrates, not refined white flour. If they are corn starch or modified starch as in baby foods, they are just empty calories (Ballentine, 1978).

Starch is stored carbohydrate, and it feeds the plant while it is first growing. Also, it has to have protein, vitamins and minerals to help the plant grow. Grains are our major carbohydrate food (Ballentine, 1978).

FIBER

There has been a lot of publicity about the value of fiber or roughage in the diet in the last few years.

The lack of fiber in the diet is believed by some to be the primary cause of appendicitis, diverticulitis, and tumors of the colon and rectum. Fiber decreases the transit time of feces through the alimentary canal, and increases the bulk and softness of feces. The faster transit time means less contact of carcinogens with bowel walls.

One hundred percent extraction wholewheat flour contains two percent crude fiber. Seventy percent extraction has 0.1 percent fiber; the 30 percent that's removed contains most of the fiber, protein, vitamins and minerals. Millet meal contains 3.0 percent fiber (Burkitt and Trowell, 1975).

The Irish potato contains about as much fiber as wholemeal bread (5.4 g/1000 calories). It isn't true that most of the food value is in the peel. Protein in the peel is 2.5 g/100 g; inside, 2.1 g/100 g. Mature dried beans and peas have 20–30 grams of protein in 100 grams, 300–400 calories/100 g, and 4–7 g fiber in 100 grams (2–3 times as much as wholewheat bread) (Burkitt and Trowell, 1975).

In 1963 a popular idea was that "fiber is a disadvantage." This idea was common in treating all diseases of the colon, but the treatment has now been entirely reversed for many of those diseases.

Fiber acts like a sponge and soaks up cholesterol and secretes it, thus cleaning out the colon and getting rid of cholesterol that might otherwise get to the coronary vessels (Spiro, 1976). People in prosperous developed countries where food is highly refined and where people take little exercise usually should eat more fiber.

In many journal articles, physicians report that their patients may not adjust rapidly to a high-fiber diet if they've suffered from constipation for years. But they will usually adjust slowly and profit greatly from such a diet.

CHANGING COOKING HABITS

You'll probably want to try your old favorite recipes using whole grains. But with all the changes you'll have to make, they won't taste the same. However, you'll be delighted with the new recipes which are already adjusted for heavier flours and different sweeteners; there'll be no changes for you to make. So rather than trying to change your old recipes, find exciting new ones.

However, if you have a special old recipe you want to try, here are the changes you'll make. Use ¾ cup of wholewheat for each cup of white flour in your old recipe. Use only two tablespoons of butter for every three called for. You may need to use 1 or 2 tablespoons more liquid than the recipe calls for in cakes and a little more than that in bread.

When foods, including cereal grains, are browned, the amino acids may be changed into compounds which the body cannot use. In bread, the amino acid is often lysine, the one that grains are already short in. The most important thing to remember about browning is not to overdo it, especially not to burn food. Do not eat food that is burned. Minerals may be changed in form so they lose their ability to join with amino acids. If they can't join, they can't be assimilated in the body.

We should fortify all breads we make so they'll be complete proteins. Here's how.
Put in the bottom of every cup of flour:
1 T soy powder
1 T powdered milk (non-instant)
1 T wheat germ
1 T bran
Fill cup with wholewheat flour or with half and half wholewheat and unbleached flour till your family gets used to eating natural foods.

Another change we'll make is to use butter—the best fat for cooking. It's a natural saturated fat. Oils, margarines and hard white shortenings are all manmade—so processed that they're dangerous. Their chemical structure is changed so it doesn't fit the chemistry of our cells. Let's use the best kind of fat—butter.

Other hints: While dough is rising in a well-greased loaf pan, it is advisable to set pan in a warm oven. Keeping a pan filled with water in the oven during rising and baking time will make the bread rise faster and have a tender crust.

Do not keep adding flour until you have let the recommended recipe "rest." Five minutes is plenty of time. Bran absorbs moisture; if more flour is added, the loaf will be hard and heavy. When bread is done, remove from pan and allow to cool on rack. Bread will cut easier when loaf is cooled.

BASIC PROCESSOR BREAD THE EASY WAY

In a small bowl, stir to dissolve:
⅓ c warm water
1 t honey
2 t baker's yeast
Place in processor bowl and process for 15 seconds:
3 c wholewheat bread flour
1 t salt
2 t honey
2 T butter cut into small chunks
Add yeast mixture to processor and very slowly add through the chute:
up to 1 c warm water
Run the processor until the dough forms a ball on top of the blade. Stop adding water at this point. Put in an oiled bowl and cover. Let rise in warm place until double. Punch down and put in in 9×5″ inch loaf pan. Now it's time to set the oven at 350 F. Let dough rise again until double. Bake about 40 minutes.

This first recipe may change your baking habits so that you won't need any other method of making raised bread. I always thought the easy way to make bread was to make many loaves at a time. That's not as fast as one at a time, one after the other. My friend who clues me in to many new methods gave me this recipe and, nodding her head with great conviction, she said, "It's easy." I'm a believer!

I've tried several other recipes using this method. They all work well.

Variations: Replace ½ c wholewheat flour with ½ c wheat germ. Add 2 T dark brown sugar.
Or: Make hamburger buns: After the dough rises the first time, form it into a roll about 2 inches in diameter and cut it into equal slices. Pat out each slice to 4–5 inches in diameter,

let rise, and bake on foil-lined baking sheet for 15–20 minutes.

Or: Replace ½ c wholewheat flour with ⅓ c soy flour and 3 T carob powder. Add 2 T brown sugar (optional). This recipe is sticky; it doesn't make a ball on the blades, but it works well anyway. Just transfer the dough to a buttered bowl, and let it rise till double in bulk. Then turn it into a bread pan and let it rise again till double, and bake. To make this sticky dough into rolls, just pick up a small amount of dough with a rubber scraper and place it on the foil-covered cookie sheet. The dough is shaped somewhat like a crescent, so I curve the pieces around a little bit more to make them look like croissants.

You may try your favorite bread recipe; just keep to the original 3 cups of flour and approximately 1 cup of water. Add nuts, seeds, raisins or other goodies. If you use wheat germ and bran, you might prefer using 1 T yeast rather than 2 t.

If you have no processor, you can use the One-Hour, No-Hands recipe; it's next best, but Christmas is always coming. What a wonderful gift for your spouse—a food processor—to help keep him/her well.

BASIC BREAD RECIPE USING ELECTRIC MIXER

ONE-HOUR, NO-HANDS BREAD

The bread made from this recipe is a heavy, peasant-type loaf, very dense. If you like that texture, you will probably like this bread, because it has a good flavor. Some people have had trouble with it because they either heat the yeast to too high a temperature or agitate it too much. Stick to the temperatures given and to the speed given for the mixer, and it should come out just right.

Preheat in oven at 325 F for 10 minutes in large bowl of the electric mixer (if it's a metal bowl):

    1 c soy flour
    4 c wholewheat flour
    2 c wheat germ
      or 1 c wheat germ and 1 c bran

While flour is heating, place in blender (or in bowl) and blend:

    1 c warm water
    ¼ c molasses
    ½ c honey
    ¼ c melted butter
    1 T salt
    ½ c powdered milk

Blend for a few seconds, then sprinkle on top of the mixture, stir in gently with a fork, and let stand for five minutes:

    3 T dry yeast

Remove flour from oven. Add blender mixture to flour mixture with two more cups of warm water. Mix in electric mixer at low speed for two minutes. Scrape from beaters and bowl into buttered pans—one 9 × 5″ or two 7 × 3 × 2″.

Place pan in warm place to rise for 10 minutes or more, covered with a towel. Bake at 350 degrees F for 25 or 30 minutes for small loaves, up to 50 minutes for large loaf.

Make rolls or hamburger buns. You may need to add more flour to make the rolls stand up. Roll into balls in your hands, flatten out on buttered cookie sheet. Brush with melted butter, cover with waxed paper and let rise. Experiment with the amount of flour you like. Most flours differ. This method can be used with any recipe. The dough can be sticky or rather stiff. Stiff dough winds around the beaters, sometimes around just one beater. Nothing seems to make any difference in the breads—they all taste all right.

If this bread is too sweet, just cut down the sweetener to one tablespoon of either honey or molasses.

The top of the dough usually smooths out while rising and baking. The top may be left plain, dusted with flour, or glazed with milk for a shiny crust. A saltwater glaze gives a crisp, hard crust. The loaf may be sprinkled with cracked wheat, sesame seeds or poppy seeds. If you like a hard crust, put water in a shallow pan in the bottom of the oven. The texture of the bread is improved.

The oven must be preheated. Bread is done

when it shrinks slightly from the sides of the pan. Cool the loaf on a wire rack.

CORNELL BREAD

Cornell bread was invented by Dr. Clive M. McCay of Cornell University. It may be a nice way to break your family in on good bread if they won't accept 100 percent wholewheat at first.

Heat in 350 F oven 10 minutes:
    5 c flour (part unbleached, part wholewheat)
    1 T sea salt
    2 T wheat germ
Place in large bowl of electric mixer:
    3 c warm water
    2 T honey
    2 T dry yeast
Let stand until yeast bubbles up (5–10 minutes). Add:
    warm flour mixture
    ⅜ c soy powder
    ⅜ c non-instant powdered milk
    2 T melted butter
Mix at low speed in electric mixer for about two minutes, until the dough gets stretchy. Place in two 7×3×2″ or one 9×5″ buttered pan. Let rise in warm place about 10 minutes. Bake at 350 F for 30 minutes or so.

RAISIN BREAD

Follow the method for making One-Hour, No-Hands bread.

Dry ingredients in oven:
    1 t salt
    4 c wholewheat flour
Liquid ingredients in blender:
    ⅓ c melted butter
    ½ c honey or dark brown sugar
    1 c raisins
    4 eggs
    1 c water
Stir in with a fork and let stand about 10 minutes:
    2 T dry yeast
Mix as in basic recipe. Mix in a cup 1 T dark brown sugar and 1 t cinnamon. Dribble the

mixture over the dough as it beats during the last two or three seconds. Bake by basic recipe.

EASY FRENCH BREAD

This bread is made by a different, easier method of kneading. This method might work for all breads; I'll try them some day. For now, try this and see if you like it.

Set oven at 375 F. Mix lightly in a large bowl; let sit until the yeast bubbles:
    2 c warm water
    2 T honey
    1 T dry yeast granules
Add and beat well with a spoon, then cover and set in a warm place to rise:
    2 T melted butter
    2 t sea salt
    4½ c wholewheat flour
        or enough to make a thick batter
At 10-minute intervals stir and "knead" the dough with a spoon five more times. This takes just a minute or two. Then turn the dough out on a plate and cut it in half. Make two balls, cover with a damp towel and let it rest for 10 minutes. Put the dough in two buttered 7×3×2″ pans and allow to rise till double, brush with cold water and sprinkle with sesame seeds if you wish. Bake for 35 to 40 minutes. Scoot a piece of butter around on top of the loaves while still warm to make a nice crust.

ANGEL FOOD BREAD

My husband has always said that my cakes taste like bread and my breads taste like cake. But the first time I made this recipe, he called it "Angel Food Bread." I think he chose the right name, so that's what I'm calling it. It is adapted from a brioche recipe.

Set oven at 350 F. Mix in small bowl in order given:
    ¼ c warm water
    ½ t honey
    1 T dry yeast
Scald ½ c milk and set aside to cool to luke-warm. In mixer, cream:
    1 c butter
    ⅓ c brown sugar or honey
    ½ t salt

Add yeast and milk to butter mixture in bowl.
Add and mix well:
1 egg yolk
3 whole eggs
4 c wholewheat flour
Beat in mixer on low speed for 10 minutes or
until dough clears the sides of bowl. Dough
will be stretchy.

Spoon dough into well-buttered muffin pans or
into a shallow loaf pan about 6×9″. Cover and
let rise until double. Brush with one beaten
egg white mixed with 1 T brown sugar. Bake
about 30 minutes. The topping tastes good when
this bread is eaten fresh, but it doesn't freeze
well.

MAKING MUFFINS

When you make cookies, muffins, or other
baked products, keep the flours, baker's yeast,
bran, wheat germ, soy powder and powdered
milk in a bicycle basket in the freezer. Take
the basket to the kitchen counter. A trip to the
fridge for butter, milk and eggs, and you're
ready to start.

Open up the bags of dry ingredients. They
don't have to be taken out of the basket. Don't
sift the flour; fluff it in the bag with a long-
handled measuring cup, then measure. The best
flour is fresh ground. Try to find a source—
maybe someday you'll want to buy a mill. Dump
all the dry ingredients in a bowl. Dump the
liquids in the blender. Stir and buzz both; pour
the liquids into the dries. If you're making
muffins, mix just until the flour disappears. If
you work a long time at it, the muffins will be
tough. Turn the batter into a 9×9×1″ pan.
Bake at 400 F. Square pans are easier to wash
than round muffin pans—we save a minute
here and a minute there. Square muffins taste
just as good as round ones. Start mixing another batch immediately. Don't wash the bowl
and blender between recipes—no one minds if
a little cornmeal gets in the bran muffins. At
least, I haven't had any complaints, and we
save three or four minutes each time.

When all the muffins and breads are cooked
and cool, cut in squares. Split each square and
store in freezer. When ready to eat, warm in
toaster oven. The split muffins are thin enough
to thaw quickly. I can make six different kinds
of muffins, biscuits or quick breads in 30
minutes. That's enough for a month for my
family of two and some for the rest of the
family when they come to visit.

Not all the muffins are cooked and out of the
oven in 30 minutes, but I am out of the kitchen.
I set the timer and go back and switch pans
from time to time, but we can't count that
cooking time.

MY FAVORITE:
WHEAT GERM MUFFINS

Heat oven to 400 F. Place dry ingredients in
bowl:
1 c wholewheat pastry flour or part cornmeal or oat flour
½ t sea salt
3 t baking powder
¼ c powdered milk (non-instant)
1 c wheat germ (or half bran)
Place liquids in blender:
1 c milk
2 eggs
2 T butter melted in pan you'll cook muffins
in
½ c raisins (chopped dates, nuts, coconut,
ground dried apricots, diced raw apple—
your choice)
Turn into 9×9×1″ pan. Bake at 400 F 15–20
minutes.

Or: Swirl spoonfuls of pureed fresh fruit or
soaked dried fruit at intervals into batter in
the pan.

SOYA MUFFINS

Place in mixing bowl:
½ c non-instant powdered milk
pinch salt
1 T orange rind
¾ c soy flour or powder
¾ c wheat germ
Whirl in blender:
3 egg yolks
3 T honey
½ c raisins

1 T melted butter
1 c sweet or sour milk
Add to blender mix and chop:
  ½ c nuts
Add blender mix to bowl mix; stir lightly. Beat and fold in:
  3 egg whites beaten stiff but not dry
Bake at 325 F for 25 minutes.
Turn into a 9×9×1″ pan.

CORN MUFFINS

Heat oven to 425 F. Mix in bowl:
  ¾ c wholewheat flour
  ¾ c stone ground cornmeal
  2 t baking powder
  ¾ t salt
  2 T sunflower seeds powdered in blender
Mix in blender:
  2 eggs
  ¾ c milk
  2 T butter melted in 9×9×1″ pan you'll bake
    muffins in
Pour liquids over solids and stir quickly until flour is gone. Place the batter in the hot buttered pan. Bake about 25 minutes.

SUNFLOWER SEED SQUARES

Heat oven to 300 F. In blender, mix to a powder:
  1 c sunflower seeds
  ½ c wheat germ
  ½ c rolled oats
  1 T orange rind
Transfer to bowl. Separate 4 eggs. In blender, combine and mix, but don't pulverize nuts and fruit:
  4 egg yolks
  ½ c coconut
  segments of one large orange (remove
    membrane)
  ½ c nuts
  ½ c dates or raisins
  2 T soft butter
Pour blender mix into bowl mix and blend lightly. Beat with egg beater and fold in till just blended:
  4 egg whites
Bake in 9×9×1″ pan for 35–40 minutes.

CRACKERS

Almost everybody likes crackers, and we eat them too, but we make our own. Instead of rolling them out and cutting them in shapes as the recipe says, roll the dough in a long roll as you do for ice box cookies. Then put it in the freezer overnight.

When you get it out, cut a thin slice. If it cuts well without cracking, it's thawed enough. If not, wait a few minutes and try again. There'll be a time that the dough will slice paper thin very easily. Cut all the dough fast and put it on cookie sheets or on foil cut to fit the cookie sheets. (The dull side of foil goes next to the food.) If you leave any slices to transfer later, you'll never get them up off the counter—they'll be too soft. Bake, but not too long. You may want to toast them again later, so allow for a little more browning.

When the crackers get cool, store in the fridge or freezer and get just enough out to eat at one time. They're good warmed in the toaster oven with cheese or peanut butter. You can make up your own cracker recipes. Just use a drop cookie recipe, omitting the baking powder and eggs and most of the sugar, too. Continue the recipe as above.

To make different shapes, try flattening the roll and making a square. It will have rounded corners, but that's all right. Or flatten it until the slices will be in the shape of bars, about 1″ by 3″.

Another method which I call crackers is to make a muffin recipe, turn it out into a large pan about 9×12 inches, and bake. It will be thin. Cut into squares when done, then when cool, split each square. Freeze in a plastic bag. To serve, put the split squares in the toaster oven. They aren't exactly like crackers, but they're close to it, and they really are good, especially when made with corn meal.

My favorite cracker is made by a recipe I offered to the listeners once during a radio call-in program. I spread the dough on cookie sheets, put another sheet on top of the first, put both on the floor and jump up and down on the top tray. Hundreds of listeners wrote and asked for my jump-on crackers, so that's what I call them, too. Here's the recipe in detail.

JUMP-ON CRACKERS

This recipe is adapted from *Laurel's Kitchen: A Handbook for Vegetarian Cookery and Nutrition*, by Laurel Robertson, Carol Flinders, and Bronwen Godfrey, copyright 1976 by Nilgiri Press, Petaluma, CA 94952. The original name for the recipe was Graham Crackers.

Place in food processor and process for about 1 minute:

    2 c wholewheat flour
    ½ c unrefined wheat bran
    ½ c raw wheat germ
    1 t baking powder
    ½ t baking soda
    ¼ t sea salt

Add and mix to the consistency of coarse meal:

    ½ c butter (1 stick) cut into ½ inch slices

Add and mix to the consistency of sticky crumbs:

    ½ c whole milk

When you pinch the dough between your fingers, it sticks together, but it doesn't stick to your fingers.

Cover two old TV trays with foil—dull side next to the food. Sprinkle ½ the sticky crumbs on each tray. Pat out as evenly as you can. Place another sheet of foil on top of the dough. Place another tray on top of each tray, one at a time. Put the two trays, stacked on top of each other on the floor. Jump up and down on the top tray. The crumbs will spread out smooth and thin. Let your children or grandchildren do the jumping. They'll love helping you make crackers. Peel off the foil, score to make whatever size cracker you wish, prick with a fork, bake at 350 degrees F for 10 to 12 minutes.

If you get the dough too wet, it will be hard to spread out. If it is too dry, it will not hold together after it is cooked.

The original recipe says roll the dough out directly on the cookie sheet and cut into squares. The easiest thing to roll it with is a six-inch piece of broomhandle. But the jumping is faster and makes the crackers thinner.

If you don't have a food processor, cut the shortening into the flour mixture. Add milk, stir till you get the sticky crumbs. Continue with the recipe.

Keep these crackers handy for the children. With peanut butter, they have complete protein.

The crackers are delicious without any sugar at all. I usually make two or three recipes at a time (one after the other) and freeze them, then warm them up later in the toaster oven. My granddaughters enjoy "decorating" the crackers after they've been jumped on. Chopped nuts, coconut, carob chips and raisins all make good decorations.

CRISPY-CHEWY CORN CHIPS

Preheat oven to 400 F. Mix together in bowl:

    1 c corn meal
    ¼ c wholewheat flour
    ¼ c sesame seeds
    ¼ t salt
    ¼ t baking soda

Add and mix well:

    ¼ c butter melted in
    1 c hot tap water
    1 T cider vinegar
    1 t dark brown sugar

Let batter stand 30 minutes to thicken slightly. Drop by teaspoonfuls on foil-covered pan. Bake 8 to 10 minutes. These are best when very thin. The edges are brown and crisp, but the centers are chewy. You might want to add a little water to the batter left in the bowl. It thickens as it stands.

Yield: about 9 dozen 1″ chips.

CORN DODGERS

Mix well:

    2 c cornmeal
    1 t salt
    1 ½ c boiling water
    3-4 T melted butter
    ¼ c peanut flour (to make peanut flour, grind toasted peanuts in blender or seed mill)
    2 T sesame seeds

Drop by spoonfuls on foil-covered baking sheet. Bake about 20 minutes at 400 F.

Yield: about 2 dozen 2 to 3″ Dodgers.

BISCUITS

Wholegrain biscuits are so good in so many ways we should always have a supply in the freezer. Eat them plain with butter or topped with fresh or organically-grown dried fruit puree rather than store-bought jelly or preserves. Also they serve as the high protein base for "shortcake" topped with any creamed protein dish such as eggs, tuna, cheese and vegetable combinations or bean puree. Top them with any fruit and whipped topping for a desert that builds health. Serve the dessert about three hours after dinner for an evening snack.

I usually make three or four recipes, one after the other, and store them in the freezer. Pat them out lightly in an 8×8 or 9×9″ pan, cook them in one piece, and cut them in big squares, about 3×3″ after they're cooked and cooled. If you cut the dough before you cook it, the movement of the knife pinches the sides of the biscuits together, and they won't rise as they should.

VERSATILE BISCUITS

Set oven at 425 F. Mix in processor (steel blade) for a minute or two:
  2 c wholewheat pastry flour (or bread flour)
  2 t baking powder
  ½ t salt
  ¼ t baking soda
Add and process to a coarse meal:
  4 T cold butter
Pour meal into bowl and add all at once:
  ¾ c buttermilk or sweet milk with 2 t vinegar
If you don't use a food processor, mix the dry ingredients together with a fork, cut butter in with a pastry cutter or with two knives. Pour in milk and stir lightly. Let stand a few minutes. Stir with a rubber spatula as if you were kneading the dough. It must be handled lightly, but it won't stick together after it's cooked unless you lightly knead it. Pat into greased pan and bake for about 15 minutes.
Yield: 9 biscuits about 3″ square.

Or: Use 6 T of cold butter, process until the butter is about the size of peas. Add 2 T honey or dark brown sugar or date sugar (optional).

Or: Add 4 T sugar and 2 more T butter to dry ingredients for a super shortcake.

Or: Add nuts and raisins, dates or lightly steamed dried apricots or apples.

Or: Add 2 T sugar and ¼ t each cinnamon and nutmeg.

SUNFLOWER SEED BISCUITS

Set oven at 375 F. Grind to powder in blender or processor:
  ½ c sunflower seeds
Place in bowl, add, and mix well:
  ½ c wholewheat flour
  2 t baking powder
  ¾ t sea salt
  2 T soft butter
Add with a few quick strokes:
  ⅓ c milk
Pat lightly into greased 9″ square pan and bake 10–12 minutes.
Yield: 9 biscuits about 3″ square

PANCAKES

Probably most people don't realize how healthful pancakes can be—when we make them ourselves from scratch with healthful ingredients. The pancakes are easy to make and delicious. The main difference is that we use wholegrain flour, and we don't use syrup. You'll notice in this section the many delightful toppings for the cakes and waffles as well. Usually we have pancakes on Sunday nights, and I really look forward to those meals.

CORNMEAL PANCAKES

Dry ingredients in bowl:
  1½ c coarse cornmeal
  ½ c powdered milk
  1 t salt
  2 t baking powder
Blend liquids in blender:
  1½ c milk
  2 egg yolks
  2 T melted butter
Stir quickly, and fold in:
  2 stiffly beaten egg whites
Bake on hot griddle.
Yield: about 8 pancakes

BUCKWHEAT CAKES

Mix in a bowl:
  ¾ c buckwheat flour
  ¼ c wholewheat flour
  2 t baking powder
  ½ c wheat germ
  2 T honey
In blender, mix:
  2 eggs
  3 T melted butter
Pour liquids in measuring cup and add milk to make 1½ cups. Blend well and pour over dry ingredients. Mix lightly and cook on a large skillet or griddle.
Yield: about 8 pancakes

EASY WHEAT PANCAKES

In a bowl, mix:
  1 c wholewheat flour
  ½ t sea salt
  1 t baking soda
  1 T dark brown sugar
In blender, mix well:
  1 c sour milk or sweet milk
  1 egg
  1 T melted butter
Cook on large griddle. I often quadruple this recipe and cook plenty of cakes for the freezer. They warm up nicely in the toaster oven.
Yield: about 6 pancakes

PANCAKE TOPPINGS

FRUIT TOWER: Blend fresh or home-frozen raw peaches, plums or bananas with a little yogurt or milk to a smooth or chunky mixture. Spread between and on top of pancakes. Add a spoonful of cottage cheese to the top and sprinkle with chopped nuts. Garnish with a strawberry.

RAISIN-COCONUT SPREAD: Blend ½ c raisins and ½ c fresh coconut shreds; moisten with milk or blend with fresh fruit in season.

DATE-APPLE SPREAD: Blend 1 c dates, pitted and chopped, with 2 tart apples, chopped.

DATE-NUT SPREAD: Blend ½ c dates, pitted, with ½ c nuts, ½ c milk and about ¼ c powdered milk.

To freeze pancakes, pack the cooled cakes in plastic bags. They'll stick together, but just twist a knife blade between them, and they pop apart easily. Warm in toaster oven.

COOKED CEREAL

Grains from the health food store take longer to cook, but we don't want to spend all our time in the kitchen, so we find short cuts.

Here's the quickest way to cook cereal. The night before, place ½ c grains in a wide-mouth thermos bottle that has a plastic liner. Add 1 c boiling water. Put the top on the thermos. Swish it around a little to mix it, and let it sit on the counter all night. In the morning, your breakfast will be waiting; the grains will still be slightly warm. The pint sized thermos which holds ½ c of grain makes enough for two large servings.

Another way to speed up cooking cereal is to put ½ c of grains in a saucepan with 1 c water. Leave it on the stove to soak all night. In the morning turn the burner on, and the grain will cook in about five minutes because the cellular structure will be softened by soaking. You may have to stir it once or twice. Add raisins or other fruits, fresh or dried.

Cook according to directions on the label any wholegrain cereal, flakes, berries, etc.

millet	corn grits
cracked wheat	oat flakes
bulgur	steel cut oats
buckwheat	Scotch oats
triticale	brown rice

If the cooking instructions aren't on the label of the package you buy, see p. 61 for a cooking chart. Breakfast grains are usually a little more moist than the same grains used for lunch and supper. Vary the amounts of water to please your family.
Yield: 1 c grain and 2 c water yields about 4 servings

QUICK SPECIAL CEREAL

Serve any cooked cereal with one or more of the following:
    any fresh or home-frozen fruit
    2 T whole flaxseed
    2 T raisins
    2 T wheat bran
    2 T almonds soaked in ice water a few minutes, then chopped

FORTIFIED BREAKFAST CEREAL

Here's a way to get a complete protein and a delicious breakfast. Use 1 c of one or more of the following:

    steel-cut oats   cracked wheat
    oatmeal   brown rice
    millet   hulled barley

Cook for 30 minutes in:
    2½ c water
Add more water if needed. Three minutes before serving, stir in:
    2 to 4 T non-instant powdered milk
Yield: 4 servings

Cook a large amount of any grain in water or milk. Freeze breakfast-size portions. To thaw, put enough for breakfast in the steamer when you go into the kitchen in the morning to get your first glass of water. The grain will be thawed and ready to eat when you come back.

Or, take the grains out of the freezer the night before. Leave in the fridge overnight; they will warm up quickly in the morning.

QUICK BUT GOOD CEREAL

Place in pan and boil 5 minutes, stirring occasionally:
    1 T wholewheat flour
    2 T whole flaxseed
    1 handful raisins
    2 T wheat bran
    2–3 chopped figs
    1 c water
Serve immediately with milk or applesauce.
Yield: 2 servings

KASHA—BREAKFAST BUCKWHEAT GROATS

Bring to a boil in a heavy utensil:
    2 c water
    1 t vegetable salt
Stir and boil for one minute:
    1 c whole buckwheat groats (kasha)
Turn heat to low and simmer for 15 minutes or until all liquid is absorbed and every grain separate.
Yield: 4 servings

Kasha can also be served as a vegetable, plain or with a little gravy, in soups, in a casserole with vegetables, or sprinkled with cheese. Of course, it makes an excellent breakfast.

GRANOLA BREAKFAST COMBINATIONS

To prepare a special breakfast of dry cereal quickly and easily, keep on hand in the freezer a mixture of nuts and grains that your family likes. Serve with milk or nut milk as dry cereal. Add any fresh fruit you wish. To make nut milk, blend to a powder ¼ c of any kind of nuts. Add ½ to 1 c water and blend till smooth. This breakfast is always "special."

Grains (toast 15 minutes at 350 F)
    rolled oats
    wheat flakes
    triticale flakes
    soy flakes
    wheat germ (raw)

Nuts (raw or lightly toasted, coarsely chopped)
    almonds   pecans
    cashews   hazelnuts
    walnuts   coconut
    peanuts—always toasted

Seeds
    sesame seeds
    sunflower
    poppy

Dried Fruits
    raisins   apricots
    dates   figs

Fresh Fruits
apples   pears
bananas   peaches
apricots   cantaloupe
berries

GRANOLA

Here's a typical granola recipe.
Heat in large heavy saucepan:
½ c honey
1 T vanilla
½ c water
Add and stir well, then toast in oven at 350 F:
2 c wheat flakes or triticale
2 c soy flakes
1 c wheat germ
3 c oat flakes
½ c sesame seeds
1 c unsweetened grated coconut
Add any other grains, nuts and seeds your family likes. The cereal will begin to toast in about 15 minutes. Stir every 5 to 10 minutes

till lightly toasted. Remove from oven and immediately pour into a bowl to cool. Pour into plastic bags and freeze.
Yield: about 10 cups

Variations: If you like nutty granola, use more nuts; if you want it crunchier, leave it in the oven longer; if too crunchy, don't cook it so long. If you want more protein, use more dry milk, wheat germ and soy granules or flakes. Chopped soy nuts are good; dried pineapple is a good sweetener.

Or: Add ½ c carob powder.

With these extra proteins, a cup of granola has as much protein as two eggs and a glass of milk. That's 20 grams (*Prevention*, 1978).

An added incentive for eating granola is to serve it with either yogurt or cottage cheese or both, and it adds to the protein value.

10

VEGETABLES

BASICALLY

It's probably safe to say that most people need to add more vegetables to their diet. Especially, now, since the American Cancer Society is suggesting that we eat vegetables that contain beta-carotene to help prevent cancer. Beta-carotene is a source of vitamin A, one of the most important preventives of cancer. Vegetables can be used as main dishes (that means the protein dish) if milk and cheese sauces are added. Milk and cheese are allowed in small amounts on the cancer-prevention diet. Buttermilk makes a good base for sauce—it's already pretty thick, and its tartness goes well with vegetables. Sliced hard cooked eggs go well on vegetables and so do seeds and nuts. Broccoli, peas and cauliflower are especially good with almonds, walnuts, or cashews.

How good are commercial frozen vegetables? Not so good. They may wait around the packing plant for several days before being frozen. While waiting, they may be sprayed with chemicals to prevent spoiling and to keep away insects. Next, they're blanched to destroy enzymes; the blanching also destroys vitamins. Some vegetables, especially dark green ones, are soaked in a chemical that destroys zinc. If zinc is left in the vegetables, the color changes to a dull gray-green when the vegetables are cooked. They're not as beautiful, but they're more healthful. Tests of frozen foods by Henry A. Schroeder showed that 40-60 percent of vitamin B complex was destroyed in the freezing process.

Sometimes frozen vegetables defrost and are refrozen one or more times while in storage. This destroys vitamins and minerals and some-times the vegetables spoil. If vegetables are frozen after being sliced or chopped, they lose more food value. The best is to freeze your own vegetables as near whole as possible.

Don't buy packages of frozen vegetables that are limp, wet, sweating or covered with frost. Don't buy frozen vegetables in sauce—too many additives. Don't buy frozen beets, potatoes or carrots; they're treated with a caustic lye bath. Canned vegetables are treated, too (Goldbeck, 1973).

Canned vegetables have even less food value than frozen, and usually much less taste. The canning process causes great loss of nutrients because of its high heat. Many chemicals are added to canned vegetables, often extra acids, but occasionally baking soda is added, which destroys B vitamins. Schroeder's tests showed that from 60 to 80 percent of vitamin B complex is destroyed in canning. Canned vegetables are also soaked in a chemical that preserves color.

Probably the most damaging additive is salt. Tremendous amounts can be added, up to 4,500 percent in green beans. Sugar can be added without being stated on the label. Much of the vitamin and mineral content in canned vegetables is in the liquid, which is usually discarded. Canned vegetables are best eliminated from the diet, as are instant potatoes (Goldbeck, 1973).

Fresh vegetables at the produce counter aren't perfect, but they're usually the best we can get. They're often waxed to appear shiny—the wax isn't healthful. They can be colored. This information should be on the shipping carton, and the produce manager in the store is supposed to display a sign saying that the vegetables are artificially colored, but many don't bother to do it.

Sometimes we see sprouts on potatoes and onions. Don't buy them; they're old. Sometimes they're old but don't have sprouts because antisprouting agents have been used. That's bad, too. These agents cause cancer in mice. The amounts that humans get when they eat potatoes is about eleven times more than the dose in the mice. The investigators who reported this study suggested that the sprouting inhibitor, maleic hydrazide, should be banned (Hunter, 1971).

Some nutritionists say to peel vegetables to cook or to eat raw. That's because they are so heavily sprayed. Others say that much of the pesticide is taken up in the roots and goes to every cell in the plants, so we'll be eating the pesticide anyway. We can soak raw vegetables in a dishpan full of water with two teaspoons of chlorine in it, then soak in clear water to remove the chlorine. Some vegetables can be soaked in dish detergent, then in clear water to remove the detergent. Whichever way you clean your vegetables, if you take food supplements, you'll help keep your liver healthy enough to detoxify the poisons.

FREEZING VEGETABLES

When you freeze your own vegetables, you don't have to blanch them. They just need to be cleaned, packed whole, or cut up if you wish. They have more vitamins and minerals if left in big pieces, but it's more convenient to cut them sometimes.

Try the following just cut up or whole, without blanching or steaming (Nusz, 1972).
CELERY: cut stalks and tops
CABBAGE: cut up, or outer leaves whole for cabbage rolls
ONIONS: small whole, cut up, or tops
CUCUMBER: either whole unpeeled, sliced or diced
PEPPERS: red or green, whole or cut
PARSLEY OR LEAVES OF ANY KIND: cut up
RHUBARB: cut before packing
TOMATOES OR PEAS: anything that has a skin or peeling can be frozen whole, as peas in the pod

CORN: take off the roughest leaves and the tip of the tassel and freeze as soon as possible after picking. Let it defrost for several hours and roast it on open oven racks still in the husks at 400 degrees F until the husks are all charred dark brown. You can fix it any other way you like—steamed is also good (Nusz, 1972).

Refrigerate greens like kale, spinach, broccoli and turnip greens in the crisper or in plastic bags with holes in them for air circulation. Cucumbers, eggplants and peppers should not be put in plastic bags—they get soft.

Leave lima beans and green peas in the pod till you're ready to cook them.

Potatoes shouldn't be prepared ahead. As much as half of the vitamin C is lost by the second day. It's best to cook potatoes in their skins and eat the peeling.

Outer leaves of lettuce have more calcium, iron and vitamin A than inner leaves. Broccoli leaves have more vitamin A than flower buds or stalks. Cook and serve leaves, too.

Don't cut lettuce; it browns easily. Tear it gently. Cut carrots into quarters instead of slices. French-slicing green beans causes loss of nutrients. Using any utensil containing copper causes loss of color.

We should eat both steamed and raw vegetables each day—they're the next best food to grains, nuts and seeds. Don't reheat leftover cooked vegetables; serve cold in salad. It's best to prepare only enough vegetables for one meal.

SELECTING VEGETABLES

It may be difficult to select good vegetables. Here are some suggestions from vegetable experts.

ONIONS: The sweetest onions are Gran X and Gran O. The "O" is a yellow onion which looks like a turnip. It is round and large. Purple onions are sweetest, but some purple are the hottest grown—be careful. Pink onion is sweet but hard to get.
ENGLISH PEAS AND OKRA: buy small, tender ones that bend and are soft.
CUCUMBERS: the smaller the vegetable, the smaller the seeds. Buy green colors—no yellow.

GREEN BEANS: should snap, not bend.

TOMATOES: flavorful ones will not have a film that comes up when you scratch the skin. Those are immature. Seeds should be large. Pear-shaped tomatoes are low in acid and have a good flavor.

CARROTS: buy organically grown. Cut off ½ inch of green tip.

AVOCADOS: rough skin, Hass, are best. Fuerte have smooth, dull skin; Texas organic avocados are smooth, shiny and really good.

Vegetables are super made into soup. For smooth cream soups, blend half the vegetables in the blender with part of the stock. Transfer to a saucepan to heat. Sauté the rest of the vegetables and add to the saucepan; cook until tender. In the blender, combine milk powder with water, using a wire whisk. Add to saucepan.

Spices make good seasonings, as do dried powdered vegetables. If you like all spices in one jar, such seasonings are available at health food stores. If you use salt, use iodized sea salt or vegetable salt from health food stores.

Cook green vegetables in milk or cream sauce as follows: Prepare 1 to 1½ cups of thick cream sauce. Cut any kind of green into ¼ inch shreds. Add greens to sauce and stir until all leaves are covered with sauce. Simmer for 8 minutes, stirring occasionally. If not thin enough, add a little milk (Davis, 1947). Don't add salt. Most people salt everything anyway, and those that don't want salt will be grateful. Top cooked and raw vegetables with sesame seeds or toasted sunflower or pumpkin seeds.

Sometimes try soaking raw sunflower seeds in cold water for about ½ hour. Drain and sprinkle on raw salads or steamed vegetables. They're crisp and crunchy.

Never soak vegetables. Wash quickly in cold water. Pat dry with turkish towels. Never cut until the last minute. Don't cut with a copper knife; vitamin C is destroyed almost immediately (Walczak, 1977).

Steam vegetables in two tablespoons of water in "waterless" cookware or in a heavy pan with a heavy, close-fitting top. Best of all is a steamer with no holes in the bottom. Holes around the top let in the steam (See Kitchen Aids, p. 137). If you use waterless cookware, use high heat for one minute, reduce to simmer. Always have one burner on an electric stove turned to low so you can transfer the pan to low heat.

Vegetables can be steamed, pressure cooked, sautéed, broiled or baked. When half cooked, add a cream sauce to which are added powdered milk, cheese and/or wheat germ. Or simmer in milk and use the milk. Or cook in very little water and use the water. Dice, shred or slice vegetables; they cook faster and lose fewer nutrients. Prepare and cook just before serving.

If the fresh produce isn't fresh, use frozen vegetables. Frozen foods usually start with fully ripe vegetables.

TO COOK OR NOT TO COOK VEGETABLES

When plant foods are cooked, the heat causes the starch inside the cell to swell. This breaks the cellulose wall of the plant cell and the contents spill out so they can be digested. But some nutrients are destroyed by the heat, especially vitamin C. When the cell contents are exposed to the air, they spoil quickly, so cooked food won't keep for a long time.

The vegetables are often more easily digested because cooking breaks the long chains of molecules down to simple molecules the cells can use. Moderate heat is best. If the heat is too high, protein molecules are damaged so the amino acids are destroyed and can't be released by enzymes.

In some green leafy vegetables there are strong irritants which are broken down or removed by cooking. Raw onions cause face and eyes to burn, and we might not be able to think well for a short time after eating them.

It is thought that when man began to cook his food, the shape and size of his jaws became smaller; he could speak better and communicate better because he didn't have to have such big jaws to chew with. Some anthropologists think that cooking food is one of the most important factors in human evolution (Ballentine, 1978).

We can eat more food if it's cooked than if it's raw. The vegetables cook down, have less bulk and are more tender. The vitamins and minerals are more concentrated and more available. We can't say that all foods should be cooked or for how long. It depends on the food and on the person eating it. If he is active in his way of life, he can tolerate more raw food (Ballentine, 1978).

POTATOES AND OTHER TUBERS

Potatoes are grown to ship well; the taste is not so important. As many as one in five potatoes is damaged by mechanical harvesting. They are also damaged when washed and packed in plastic bags because the atmosphere inside the bag is too humid. Their bruises turn black and have to be cut away. We should never eat potatoes with green skins because of the poison solanine, caused by exposure to light.

Potatoes are very starchy, which is good because the starch furnishes energy for all our cells, including the brain. They have a little protein, and just under the skin are the vitamins and minerals. If a person ate all his calories in potatoes, he would get 40 grams of protein, 14 mg. of iron, 180 mg. of calcium, 34 mg. of B3, and 720 mg. of vitamin C in one day. We can't live on potatoes, but it is rather surprising that the lowly potato has all that food value.

At a luncheon one time, I naturally got started talking about nutrition. When one of the men saw me eating potatoes, he said, "How can you be a nutritionist and eat potatoes?" I was happy to tell him how healthful potatoes are, but this incident shows how little the average American knows about food. Of course, he was eating white rolls, drinking gallons of coffee and eating a plastic dessert, but he had evidently heard that potatoes have starch in them, and he thought it was bad. Potato starch is an excellent complex carbohydrate.

Sweet potatoes are no relation to white potatoes, but they are also excellent food. They are popular in the southern states. One of my nutrition students says he makes milk shakes with sweet potatoes and milk. Another says she eats sweet potatoes as dessert.

Other good tubers are Jerusalem artichokes, which look like twisted potatoes but are much

sweeter. When eaten raw they taste like water chestnuts.

Most root vegetables taste better when they're very young and tender. Young white turnips have a subtle flavor, but when turnips get bigger, they can be used in stews because they take on the flavor of whatever they're cooked with.

Kohlrabi and rutabagas are good when eaten small. Parsnips, carrots, and beets are the sweetest roots.

The greatest concentration of carotene (provitamin A) is in the skin of carrots and just under it. Don't scrape carrots—just scrub well.

ONIONS AND GARLIC

Onions have a great reputation. They are said to cure boils, restore bad eyesight, reduce blood pressure, clean out the bowels, induce sleep and lower cholesterol.

Onions need sun to ripen them, but the greater the heat, the milder the onion will taste. The mild varieties are usually sold as Bermuda onions. Red onions have a stronger flavor. Onions grown in cooler climates are smaller, stronger-flavored, and keep better. It's hard to have a year-round supply from your own garden because they will sprout or rot in storage. Leeks are a better vegetable for a home garden. They can stay in the ground all winter and they have more of some vitamins and minerals.

Garlic has all kinds of health uses: bugs can't live in it, it is said; it eliminates round and thread worms; it reduces blood pressure in 40 percent or more of cases; and it lowers cholesterol as shown in controlled animal studies. Dishes containing garlic should not be frozen because they often develop an unpleasant flavor.

GREEN LEAFY VEGETABLES

There is a wealth of vitamins and minerals in green leafy vegetables. Vitamin A is plentiful if the leaves are green and have a lot of chlorophyll. The outer leaves of cabbage may have 50 times as much carotene as the white heart.

Steamed spinach; broccoli, especially the variety Calabrese, which has a good flavor; and kale, mainly used as animal feed, are all highly nutritious. I used to grow kale. The plants look like tiny pine trees. I planted them in the front flower bed, and people would stop while driving by to ask what they were.

Cabbage, cauliflower and brussels sprouts all have good vitamin and mineral content, but are strong flavored. Chinese cabbage is milder. All these vegetables should be steamed briefly and eaten immediately (cut an X in the bottom of brussels sprouts, they cook more quickly).

TOMATOES

Tomatoes are probably the most popular raw vegetable. Sweet Italian tomatoes are outstanding. They are the only canned vegetable worth eating. (Seddon and Burrow, 1977). Fresh tomatoes sold today are poor examples of tomatoes (which everybody knows). They are grown to be heavy and have tough skins so they'll travel well. There is a prejudice against yellow tomatoes, but they have softer skins and sweeter flesh.

CUCUMBERS

Cucumbers are rather indigestible. They can be helped by slicing them thinly, sprinkling with salt and letting them set an hour. Pour off the water and eat. (The salt obviously draws out the indigestible substances and probably much of the food value. We can enjoy cucumbers as condiments, but let's get plenty of real food value from other vegetables.)

BELL PEPPERS

Bell peppers are good when green, better when red—they're sweeter and less pungent.

SQUASH

Squash have little nourishment; pumpkins are more nourishing. Pumpkin pie is good with

its added eggs and milk, if we use very little sugar.

EGGPLANT

Eggplant has little nourishment and uses up a lot of oil when it is fried. The answer to that objection is—don't fry it, and always combine it with other more nutritious meats or vegetables to improve its food value.

COOKING VEGETABLES

If you like Chinese stir-fried vegetables, don't use hot oil. It is carcinogenic. Heat about ¼ inch of water in a skillet. Stir-fry the vegetables and after the steam comes up, cover and cook a few minutes.

SWEET AND SOUR CABBAGE

Place all ingredients in steamer and steam about 8 minutes:
 2 c shredded red or green cabbage
 1 onion, grated
 juice of one lemon
 1½ t caraway seeds
 pinch ground allspice
 2 tart apples cored and diced
 1½ T honey
 1½ T butter
 2 T raisins
Stir well and serve.
Yield: 4 servings.

CHINESE CABBAGE

Slice 3 c cabbage thin across the head. Sauté lightly in butter with a little soy sauce and parsley.
Yield: 4 servings.

CABBAGE DIFFERENTE

Shred in processor (slicer blade):
 2 c cabbage
Transfer to steamer and add:

2 T butter
¼ c raisins (optional)
¼ c wine or apple cider vinegar
¼ t salt
Yield: 4 servings.

VEGETABLES IN CREAM SAUCE

Steam 3 c chopped vegetables till tender. Make cream sauce in blender:
  1 c milk
  2 T butter
  2 T wholewheat flour or arrowroot powder
Cook in serving dish over direct heat, stirring till thick. Add drained vegetables to sauce, mix well. Add seasonings. Stir in or sprinkle on top:
  1. chopped toasted peanuts
  2. toasted almonds and thin slices of raw celery for crunch
  3. Toasted cashews sprinkled with paprika
  4. grated cheese
  5. nutmeg or thyme, sunflower seeds soaked in ice water for 30 minutes and drained (put liquid in soup kettle in freezer)

Variations: Cook in milk, or steam and add milk mixed with non-instant powdered milk.
Yield: 4 servings

GREENS QUICK-COOKED WITH MILK

Place in blender:
  1 c milk
  4 T non-instant powdered milk
Blend till smooth. Simmer milk in large saucepan with 3 c chopped greens till greens are tender. Season to taste and serve over any grains. Garnish with toasted almonds.
Yield: 6 servings

STEAMED GREENS WITHOUT MILK

Steam 3 c washed and dried chopped greens.
Seasonings:
  1. Lemon juice and sea salt
  2. Onions frizzled in butter
  3. Slice stems of heavy greens (e.g. Swiss chard) crosswise. Steam five minutes, add leaves. Garnish with a few raisins, sprinkle with toasted sunflower seeds.

4. Diced celery and green pepper, 2 T finely chopped nuts or sesame seeds, 1 t lemon juice and sea salt. Add hard-boiled eggs (optional).
Yield: 4 servings

CELERY

Celery is a favorite. It has good mineral value and is very low in calories.
Slice in processor:
  6 large ribs of celery
Steam till tender. Don't overcook
Prepare 1 c of medium cream sauce in a heatproof serving dish. Season with tarragon, nutmeg, and a bit of garlic (optional). Add celery, stir lightly, and serve.
Yield: 4 servings

GREEN BEANS

Wash well and steam:
  4 c green beans, loosely packed
Season with:
  1. sautéed mushrooms or onions
  2. toasted almonds
  3. grated Parmesan cheese
  4. diced leftover sweet potato
  5. sunflower seeds sautéed in butter, dash of garlic salt, ½ t curry powder
  6. Sunflower seeds soaked in ice water about 15 minutes and drained.
Yield: 4 servings

SUMMER SQUASH

Steam until tender:
  3 c lightly packed summer squash
Season and serve.
Seasonings:
  1. 1 small, finely grated onion
     ¼ t salt
     1 T butter
     1 t honey
  2. onions steamed in butter
     tomatoes chopped coarsely
  3. ½ clove garlic
     1 T chopped parsley
     ¼ c diced celery
     ¼ t oregano
Yield: 4 servings

FRIZZLED CARROT PATTIES

Grate in processor (steel blade):
  wholewheat bread to make 1 c dry crumbs
Remove from processor to bowl. Then grate and steam until soft:
  3 c carrots
Add and mix well:
  ½ t salt
  ½ t nutmeg
Drop carrot mixture by spoonfuls into bread crumbs, turn and coat other side; transfer to skillet containing melted butter, frizzle until golden brown. Serve immediately.
Yield: 6 servings

STEAMED CARROTS

Steam until tender:
  3 c sliced carrots
Add in steamer:
  1. chopped parsley, butter
  2. butter, sea salt, basil
  3. 2 T butter, sprinkle of powdered lemon rind
Add in serving dish:
  1. ground sesame and poppy seeds mixed
  2. dribbles of honey and chopped walnuts
  3. apple sauce and lemon juice
Yield: 4 servings

SUNCHOKES-JERUSALEM ARTICHOKES

In steamer, place 4 c chopped Jerusalem artichokes. Steam lightly; the flavor gets strong if overcooked. Season and serve:
  * Serve in cream sauce
  * Season with butter and toasted sesame seeds.
Yield: 4 servings

SWEET POTATOES

Yams are darker and sweeter than sweet potatoes. Slice either and alternate with sliced apple in baking dish. Sprinkle raisins and nuts around.
Bake several large sweet potatoes at a time uncovered in a 350 F oven for 20 minutes. Eat some while hot; freeze the rest. To serve, stir and heat in saucepan till well mixed:

leftover sweet potatoes
honey
grated orange rind
butter
chopped orange sections

Frizzle sliced sweet potatoes in butter. They taste so good, they need no additional seasoning.
Yield: allow ½ c sweet potatoes per serving

NEW POTATOES

Steam scrubbed new potatoes till barely tender.
Seasonings:
  sea salt   butter
  garlic   lemon juice
  paprika
Let sit over hot water a minute or two; serve.
Yield: allow ½ c new potatoes per serving

BAKED POTATOES

Baked potatoes are a good source of vitamin C. Serve with cream sauce with chopped spinach and/or chopped parsley, or sour milk topping (p. 28).
Yield: allow 1 average potato per serving

POTATTIES

When my children were little, we always ran the words "potato" and "patties" together and said "potatties."

Peel, cut in chunks and steam until soft:
  4 medium potatoes
Mash well and add (if you wish, transfer to processor and whip with plastic blade):
  3 T butter
  2 egg yolks
  ¼ c whole milk
  salt and pepper to taste
Spoon by ¼ cupfuls on to a buttered baking sheet and lightly brown in a 375 F oven.

Or: frizzle in a moderate skillet in butter, turning once.
Yield: 6 servings

GREEN BEAN-TOMATO COMBO

Blend into crumbs and set aside:
  2 slices homemade wholegrain bread
Snap into small pieces and steam till tender:
  2 c (½ pound) fresh green beans
Add to beans in steamer; stir till well mixed:
  salt and pepper
  2 large peeled, chopped home-frozen
    or fresh tomatoes
    or one cup peeled small tomatoes
  1 T butter
  bread crumbs
Heat through and serve with freshly grated or frozen grated cheese.
Yield: 6 servings

WINTER SQUASH

Steam acorn or other winter squash. Peel, then blend in processor (plastic blade) or blender. Season and serve. Seasonings suggested:
  * Molasses to taste, pinch salt, pinch nutmeg, yolk of one egg. Leave in steamer for 5 minutes. Sprinkle with chopped pecans and serve.
  * Mix with raisins and yogurt.
  * Serve with creamed spinach.
  * Add brown sugar, butter and cinnamon.
Yield: allow ½ c squash per serving

NUTTY ZUCCHINI

Steam until tender, not mushy:
  2 medium zucchini, sliced ½ inch thick
Add:
  2 T butter
  salt and pepper to taste
  ¼ c coarsely chopped walnuts
  ¼ t thyme
Serve immediately.
Yield: 4 servings

CHEESY ZUCCHINI-TOMATOES

Preheat oven to 350 F. Slice in thin slices:
  3 large zucchini
Blend in blender:
  6 large skinned tomatoes
Butter a casserole and arrange zucchini and tomatoes in layers with:

  1 pound mozzarella cheese, thinly sliced
  ½ pound ricotta cheese
  (last layer should be mozzarella)
Bake 45 minutes.
Yield: 8 servings

STEAMED VEGETABLE COMBINATIONS

Steam vegetables together for super stews. Remember to cook small amounts of each vegetable—we don't want to prepare more than the family can eat at one meal, because we always want to eat freshly prepared vegetables. Use your steamer or a heavy saucepan with 2 or 3 T of water in it. Here are some combinations you might like:
  potatoes, carrots and cabbage
  onions, green peppers and tomatoes
  potatoes, onions and zucchini
  onions, garlic, broccoli and carrots

Seasonings are as varied as the vegetables: cheese; butter, garlic, and bay leaf; oregano, sea salt, and pepper. Combine any vegetable and seasoning with a cup or so of leftover cooked whole grains or tofu (soy cheese), and heat 5 more minutes.
Yield: Allow ¾ c vegetables and ½ c grains per serving.

SOUPS

Soups are ideal foods. They can have more vitamins and minerals than many other foods, and taste better; so everybody likes them.

FREEZER SOUP

One of my favorites is Freezer Soup. It is made from the bits and pieces of meat and vegetables that were left over after meals the preceding month or so. The amounts were too small to make it back to the table by themselves, so they were put into the freezer pot. That is a big container with a tight-fitting top. We have the most tremendous variety in our Freezer Soups because it's different every time it is served, since leftovers are never the same. One month I had served Mexican Bean Treat, but I overestimated the number of people to eat it, and we had quite a bit left over. Nevertheless, I put it all in the freezer pot, and with the rest of the soup fixings that month, it turned out to be extra good.

Other soups are easy to prepare. Often I steam a variety of vegetables, puree about half in the blender, and add them back to the soup kettle. An extra bit of hamburger pattie or other animal protein lends its nice flavor to the mix. Seasoning is always at hand. I keep powdered vegetable seasonings from the health food store to add to the herbs and spices commonly available.

BASIC SOUP

Most soups begin about the same way. We sauté onion in butter, add green pepper or celery with a bay leaf, basil, thyme and other favorite spices. Add dried beans and peas and long-cooking whole grains such as brown rice and millet, if that's what tantalizes your taste buds today. Add 8 to 10 cups of water and bring to a simmer. Cook about 1½ hours until the dried beans and peas are almost tender, then add fresh vegetables of several kinds. If you're having just fresh vegetable soup today, add them to the sautéed onions and spices and simmer about 30 or 40 minutes until done. Add any leftover grains, beans, and meat patties, diced. Season to your taste, and serve gladly.

Of course, we add the slow-cooking vegetables first and the diced leafy greens such as spinach and parsley for the last 10 minutes or so of cooking. Test for salt at the end. If you've made enough for a crowd and there's just two of you, store the rest in meal-size portions in the freezer.

"ANY" SOUP

Prepare nut milk. Blend dry in blender:
 ½ c nuts (almonds, walnuts, sunflower seeds, cashews, peanuts or a combination)
Add and blend well:
 2½ c water
Add vegetables:

1 c carrots, tomatoes, celery, spinach, parsley, asparagus, potatoes, or a combination
Add seasonings:
 butter, kelp, vegetable broth powder, bell pepper, garlic, onion, dill, or other
Yield: 4 1-cup servings

POTATO SOUP

Place in soup kettle, bring to a boil, and simmer until potatoes are tender, about 15 minutes:
 2 c water
 4 small potatoes, peeled and cubed (about 2½ c cubed potatoes)
 1 t dill seeds, ground
 1 onion, finely chopped
 1 leek, chopped
 sea salt to taste
Puree the mixture in the blender. Mix together:
 1 T soy flour
 1 T brewer's yeast
Gradually blend in:
 1½ c milk
Reheat and serve garnished with parsley or chives.
Yield: 4 approximately 9-oz. servings

SPLIT PEA SOUP

Place all ingredients in soup kettle:
 2 c split green peas, picked over and washed
 5 c cold water
 ¼ c butter
 2 t sea salt
 2 ribs celery with leaves, chopped coarsely
 ½ white turnip, sliced
 1 onion, sliced
 1 large carrot, quartered
 1 bay leaf
 ⅓ t chervil
 ½ t savory
Bring to a boil, cover and simmer for about 2 hours or until peas are tender. Blend soup in a blender until smooth.
Yield: 8 1-cup servings

CELERY SOUP

Combine in large kettle:
 1 quart chopped celery—use the outer ribs with leaves

2 c boiling water
1 large potato, grated
Combine in a saucepan:
  2 T butter
  4 T wholegrain flour
Add slowly:
  1 quart milk, scalded
Bring the milk to a boil and stir until mixture thickens slightly. Add and stir milk into the celery mixture with:
  sea salt to taste
  ⅛ t nutmeg
Add and stir into soup:
  2 hard-boiled eggs, chopped
Serve immediately.
Yield: 8 1-cup servings

11

SALADS AND SALAD DRESSINGS

VEGETABLE SALADS

Salads are about the easiest foods to prepare. We're used to having salad every day and mostly the preparation will be the same—prepare salads at the last minute because cut vegetables lose food value fast.

Many nutritionists say eat salad last and meat first. When we eat salad first, the hydrochloric acid in the stomach will be diluted, and it won't be acid enough to digest and assimilate proteins, vitamins and minerals. When we eat meat and other proteins first, the protein gets to the stomach while the stomach acid is still strong enough to digest proteins well. Try switching to proteins first and salad last if you have any digestive problems.

What salads are best? For tossed green salads, we need dark green leaves because they have more food value than white head lettuce. Use romaine, red tip, Bibb, Boston, salad bowl, dandelion greens and other leaf lettuces. We can use spinach occasionally. We should eat as many different raw vegetables as we can get.

Keep your food processor handy to chop and slice these vegetables.

For best salads, use the freshest vegetables you can find. If you use supermarket vegetables, try to find out when deliveries are made to the store so they will be as fresh as possible. Store all vegetables unwashed and wash the amount needed for each meal. Wash quickly in three waters. Cut leaves of parsley off the stems and put leaves in the salad spinner with romaine or other leaf lettuce and celery stalks. Spin till dry. Dry smooth vegetables with a soft turkish towel. Adelle Davis (1947) says to put leafy vegetables in a cheesecloth bag or pillow case and whirl by hand or in the final cycle of an automatic washing machine. They are dry in a minute.

Put parsley leaves in the processor (steel blade) for fast, even chopping. This is the best way I've found to chop parsley. I also like to use the slicer blade and pack the feed chute tightly with celery and slice it for salad and soup.

Parsley is available most of the year, and should be used almost daily. The dark green leaves have a lot of vitamin A and other nutrients. Romaine lettuce has more than twice as much calcium, twice the iron and vitamin C, and more than four times as much vitamin A as iceberg lettuce (*Prevention*, 1978).

Serve a fast vegetable salad sometimes: cut the vegetables in sticks and pieces, serve the salad dressing in a bowl, and let each person dip his own. This saves a few minutes, and we need to save all the minutes we can. Eat the sticks and pieces with nuts or seeds, and you won't need salad dressing. In fact, this way of serving salad helps us enjoy the taste of the food much more than with an oily dressing. Fresh, crisp dark green leaves with crunchy cashews, crisp carrots with toasted peanuts, celery with pecans, or any combination of vegetables and nuts should be found more and more on our salad plates.

SALAD FIXINGS

Always keep parsley on hand and add it to every tossed salad. It has tremendous amounts of nutrients. Celery, also, should be in every tossed salad.

Here are other "additives" for peppy salads:

VEGETABLES

tomato wedges	olives
carrot sticks	cucumber
green pepper	potatoes
Jerusalem artichokes	broccoli
green beans	fresh corn kernels
cauliflower	pickled beets
fresh beets	zucchini
mushrooms	grated raw sweet
sprouts of all kinds	potatoes
cabbage	

FRUITS

orange sections	apples
tangerine sections	cherries
pineapple	pears
peaches	melons
grapes	

PROTEIN "ADDITIVES"

hard-boiled eggs	shrimp
tuna	salmon
cheese strips	strips of beef, turkey,
anchovy fillets	chicken, fish
cottage cheese	ricotta cheese

EXTRAS

basil	dill
lemon juice	sesame, sunflower,
raisins	pumpkin seeds
wholewheat toast	nuts of all kinds
cubes	dates
soy bacon bits	

GASPACHO

Here's a salad to drink. Blend a little at a time all the ingredients:
    1 small onion
    1 cucumber, chopped
    1 or 2 cloves of garlic, chopped
    ¼ c cider vinegar
    2 T soy oil
    1 bell pepper, chopped with seeds
    3 ripe tomatoes, peeled and cut in chunks
    2 t paprika
    1 raw egg
Place the puree in a pitcher and mix well. Chill. Serve cold.
Yield: 4 servings

LEAFY SALAD

Tear in bite-size pieces:
    4 large romaine leaves or combination of green
        leaves
    sliced radishes, carrots and green pepper
Dressing: Blend all together:
    1 T honey
    ¼ c sesame seeds
    ¼ apple, peeled
    pinch black pepper
    pinch dry mustard
Yield: 4 servings

SALAD COMBINATIONS

Combine and toss:
1. Zucchini, onions, parsley, dill. Dressing: lemon juice, honey, sesame seeds.
2. Leaf lettuce, thin carrot sticks, spinach, ripe olives.
    For extra protein: hard cooked egg, shrimp, turkey strips.
3. Green beans, walnuts, onions (optional), green pepper.
    Dressing: 1 t lemon juice and seasonings (fresh dill or rosemary).
4. Cabbage, fresh pineapple.
    Dressing: lemon juice, ground cashews.

RED BEAN SALAD

Drain well:
    1 c red beans
Combine with:
    2 sliced hard-boiled eggs
    1 minced onion
    1 rib chopped celery
Linda's dressing (p. 97)

Or: Instead of red beans, use lima beans combined with raw chopped onions; chopped celery; chopped, lightly steamed or raw carrots.
Yield: 4 servings.

EGG SALAD

Mix together well:
  2 chopped hard-boiled eggs
  1 t chopped chives (optional)
  1 T sliced olives
  2 T chopped parsley
  1 rib chopped celery
  paprika
Dressing:
  4 T cream and 1 t vinegar or 4 T cream and
    1 t lemon juice with ½ t mustard
Yield: 2 servings

SALAD DRESSINGS

NATURAL GREEN SALAD DRESSING

Combine, beat with fork, and chill:
  ¼ c yogurt
  ½ c cottage cheese
  ⅓ c chopped fresh parsley
  1½ T apple cider vinegar
  1½ T anchovy paste
  1½ T lemon juice
  ground pepper to taste
Makes 1½ cups

NO-OIL MAYONNAISE

Combine in saucepan, mix well and heat over very low heat till thick, stirring constantly with a wire whisk:
  2 eggs
  ¾ t salt
  ¼ t dry mustard
  ½ c milk or nut milk
  ½ t paprika
  3 T lemon juice
Remove from heat, then chill.
Yield: 1 cup

RUSSIAN DRESSING

In blender:
  1 c cottage cheese
  1 large home-frozen or fresh tomato
  1 T vinegar or lemon juice
Add hard-boiled egg to salad.
Yield: 1½ cups

SESAME SEED DRESSING

Blend in blender till powder:
  ½ c sesame seeds
Add and blend till smooth:
  1 c water
  juice of ½ lemon
  salt to taste
  ½ clove garlic or grated onion to taste
Yield: 1½ cups

TOFU DRESSING

Blend in blender till thick and creamy:
  1 c tofu (soy cheese)
  2 T tamari soy sauce
  ¼ t oregano
  ¼ c water
  1 clove garlic (optional)
  juice of half a lemon
  1 t lecithin
  ¼ t marjoram
Add if you wish, one or both:
  2 large mushrooms
  1 small tomato
Yield: 1½ cups

ITALIAN SALAD DRESSING

In blender, blend till smooth:
  ¼ c lemon juice
  1 clove garlic
  ¼ peeled, chopped apple
  salt to taste
  ¼ c water
  3 T grated Romano cheese
  pinch black pepper
  1 t honey
Yield: 1 cup

AVOCADO-YOGURT DRESSING

In blender:
    1 ripe avocado
Add quickly and blend lightly:
    ½ c tofu (soy cheese) or yogurt
    ⅛ t oregano
    1 t tamari soy sauce
Add if desired: ground or chopped nuts or seeds, lemon slices, sprouted alfalfa seeds or parsley.
Yield: 1 cup.

FRUIT DRESSING

In blender, blend lightly:
    1 c yogurt
    1½ t papaya juice or cantaloupe chunks
    3 sections fresh orange without membrane
        or ½ apple, peeled and cut into chunks
Yield: 1¼ cups

THOUSAND ISLAND DRESSING

Mix in blender:
    1 c yogurt or buttermilk combined with cottage cheese
    1 T lemon juice
    ½ t vegetable salt
    1 pimiento, chopped
    ¼ t paprika
Pour into bowl; add and mix with fork:
    ½ green pepper, chopped
    2 hard-boiled eggs, chopped
Yield: 1½ cups

GRAPEFRUIT-AVOCADO DRESSING

In blender, blend till smooth:
    1 large grapefruit, peeled and sectioned
    1 ripe avocado, peeled and diced
    1 t poppy seed
Yield: 1½ cups

VEGETABLE SALAD DRESSING

Use tofu (similar to cottage cheese but made with soy milk) in blender to cover the blades well. Add:
    onion salt or powder
    dried parsley flakes or fresh parsley

With blender running, add liquid (water or milk) or a fresh tomato, till dressing is fluffy.

Variation: Use avocado, cottage cheese, or yogurt (or any combination of the three) instead of tofu. Mix well with raw or cooked vegetables.
Yield: 1 cup

LINDA'S SALAD DRESSING

One of my nutrition friends donated this recipe when I told her I was looking for dressings without oil.

Place in blender all at once, blend till smooth, chill and serve:
    ½ c cottage cheese
    4 T Parmesan cheese
    3 T lemon juice
    ½ clove garlic
    2 coddled eggs (dipped in their shells in boiling water; four minutes for small eggs, five minutes for large)
    1½ t Worcestershire sauce
    ½ t salt
This keeps about five days in the fridge.
Yield: 1¼ cups

FRUIT SALAD DRESSING

Beat till stiff but not dry and set aside:
    3 egg whites
Beat in top of double boiler:
    3 egg yolks
    ¼ c honey
    ¼ c lemon juice
Cook, stirring till mixture thickens. Cool. Fold in egg whites.
Yield: 1¼ cups

PEANUT DRESSING

Mix with a fork:
    2 T peanut butter
    2 T lemon juice
    2 T water
Serve over banana or apple salad.

Variation: Use any ground nuts or seeds and add garlic if you wish.
Yield: 6 tablespoons

CHEESE AND TOMATO DRESSING

Blend all ingredients in blender till smooth:
- 1 c cottage cheese
- 1 fresh or home frozen tomato
- 1 T soy sauce
- ½ t thyme
- 1 clove garlic, pressed
- 1 coddled egg (dipped in boiling water for 4–5 minutes)
- 1 t lemon juice
- ½ t oregano
- 1 t vegetable salt

Yield: 1½ cups

CHEESE DRESSING

Blend all ingredients till smooth:
- 2 T Swiss, cottage, or bleu cheese
- 2 T lemon juice
- 1½ t honey
- 1 egg
- 2 T chopped parsley

Yield: ½ cup

ROQUEFORT NO-OIL DRESSING

Combine in processor (plastic blade), and mix well:
- 1 c cottage cheese
- 2 sprigs parsley or celery with leaves
- dash cayenne (optional)
- 4 oz. Roquefort or bleu cheese
- ½ c milk
- 2 T lemon juice
- ½ t salt
- ½ t tarragon

Yield: 1½ cups

APRICOT DRESSING

Blend in blender till smooth:
- ¼ c dried apricots soaked overnight and drained
- salt to taste
- ¼ lemon, seeded and peeled
- ½ c thick yogurt, cottage cheese or a mixture of both

Yield: 1 cup

KEFIR CHEESE DRESSING

Mix all ingredients well:
- 1 c kefir cheese
- ¼ t lemon juice
- 1 t honey
- ½ t salt
- ½ t paprika
- 1 t mustard
- ¼ t garlic powder

Chill and serve over a vegetable salad.
Yield: 1 cup

SESAME-AVOCADO DRESSING

Combine and mix in bowl:
- ½ c tahini (sesame seed butter)
- 1⅓ c water

Add and blend on low speed:
- ½ very large, ripe avocado, mashed
- ⅓ t cumin spice
- ½ T fresh parsley
- salt to taste

Yield: 2 cups

ZESTY SALAD DRESSING

Cook and stir till clear and thick (about 5 minutes), then cool:
- ¾ c water
- 2 t cornstarch

Place all ingredients in processor and blend till smooth:
- ¼ c vinegar (or less to taste)
- ¼ c catsup
- 1¼ t prepared mustard
- ½ t paprika
- 1 clove garlic
- 1 egg yolk
- 1 t horseradish
- ½ t salt
- ½ t Worcestershire sauce

Store in fridge, covered. Shake before using.
Yield: 1½ cups

12

FRUITS

IMPORTANCE

Fruits are important in our diet because they furnish both vitamin C and the bioflavonoids, of which there is 10 times as much in the edible part of the fruit as in the juice.

Bioflavonoids help us absorb and use vitamin C. They make the capillaries strong and make them permeable to nutrients that need to go to the cells, but they keep the substances out that should be kept out. They help keep the capillaries from rupturing and keep bacteria out of the blood so we don't get infections. People who don't have enough bioflavonoids bruise easily, with bleeding and hemorrhage.

Sources of bioflavonoids include lemons, grapes, plums, black currants, grapefruit, apricots, buckwheat, cherries, blackberries and rose hips.

Yellow fruits such as apricots, cantaloupe and persimmons are good sources of carotene which is converted to vitamin A. Apples and bananas contain fiber which is needed for bowel movements. Bananas are high in magnesium and may be useful for treatment of diarrhea, colitis, ulcers and some protein allergies. Bananas and pears are the sweetest fruits.

Fruits will lose nutrients if they are not refrigerated or if they are kept too long even if refrigerated. We should eat fresh fruits in season. Canned, dried or frozen fruits lose nutrients. Ripe fruits are best, but it's almost impossible to find them. Fruits that are not ripe should ripen at room temperature and then be stored in the fridge. Dried fruits should be soaked and then cooked about five minutes in the same water and refrigerated. Many dried fruits are better just soaked and not cooked.

We can get fresh fruit all year long—one kind or other. So let's eat fresh fruit in season and avoid canned or frozen unless we freeze it ourselves.

As for fruit juices—they're too sweet. There's as much sugar in a glass of fresh squeezed orange juice as in a glass of cola drink. Even if we drink just one glass of juice a day, we're not getting the nutrients we need because there's more to fruit than just juice. It is very likely that more and more people have diabetes partly because so many people are drinking so much fruit juice—even if no sugar is added.

There is one teaspoon of natural sugar in one medium-sized apple or orange. It takes four to six fruits to make one glass of juice which we drink quickly without thinking about our poor livers which have to store all that sugar. If we overload our livers, or if our liver cells are not working well, the cells release the sugar to the blood, and it circulates all over the body. When it goes through the pancreas, insulin pours into the blood, takes the sugar out, and stores it in the tissues. Then we don't have enough sugar in the blood, and we have hypoglycemia—low blood sugar. The first symptoms of this ailment are usually mental. We get depressed, irritable, have personality changes or fainting spells. Let's eat our fruits whole.

CHOOSING FRUITS

Here are some suggestions about selecting fruits.

CANTALOUPES: choose fruit with thick, close netting. The background should be gold or turning gold. Slight green color is all right but there should be some gold. Cantaloupes are ripe when the stem scar is smooth and the color is yellow. The blossom end should be very slightly soft. Storing cantaloupes at room temperature will soften them but not improve their flavor.

HONEYDEWS: ripe when the rind is creamy to yellowish color and has a velvety texture. Rub your hand across the melon; it should feel velvety, almost sticky. The blossom end should press in slightly, the seeds should rattle. Immature fruit is whitish-green.

WATERMELON: ripe melons have a yellow or even white color on one side. The skin is beginning to lose its shine. When thumped, it sounds hollow, but this sound is hard to determine.

ORANGE AND GRAPEFRUIT: these fruits should be heavy, with a thin skin; we should almost feel the juice inside. Rust doesn't matter on the skin. All "color added" fruits have that phrase stamped on the skin. Pink grapefruit has more than 50 times the vitamin A of white, and is usually sweeter.

PINEAPPLE: pulling leaves is not a good test for ripeness. Smell the fruit—fragrance is the easiest test; fully green fruits are all right, but the cells on the bottom should be the same size as those on the top.

MANGOS: there are twenty varieties, with the color determined by the variety. Test as for avocados—quite soft.

AVOCADOS: put in a brown paper bag to ripen, then when they are ripe, put in the fridge. In the bag, the fruit ripens fast. Sprinkle lime or lemon juice on the cut fruit to keep its color.

COCONUTS: choose a heavy one; hear the milk shake. No cracks; they cause decay inside.

TEXAS TANGERINES OR TANGELOS: not pretty, but delicious. September is the best month for these. Texas oranges are really sweet. Texas navel oranges and tangelos are supersweet. Star Ruby grapefruit are sweet, red inside, mostly seedless.

PEACHES: freestone and cling. California and Texas peaches are usually good; Texas are usually the best of all.

NUTS: there are ten kinds of pecans; they should be heavy. Small ones are often better tasting; best are Mahan, Western Schley, Stewart, Desirable.

PAPAYA: have B1, C, D vitamins; as much C as oranges.

CHERRIES: Bing are best; they should be large.

GRAPES: tart at first of season. Perlette comes in first; Thompson are better.

APPLES: Most apples bought in August have been stored since December. August's best apples are Granny Smith and winesap.

Grapes treated with gibberellic acid are plumped up 20 to 60 percent above their normal size.

If fruits or vegetables are shipped long distances, chemical preservatives can be applied directly on the fruit, or indirectly by treating the shipping container, or by incorporating the chemical in the wrapper. Toxic phenols are used (Hunter, 1971).

Phenols can destroy human chromosomes and lead to genetic mutations. To warn the consumer, a 4¾ × 2¾" card must be displayed with the fruit. But the big print says "To Maintain Freshness," which sounds as if the chemicals are improving the product. In fine print, the chemicals are listed; nowhere does the sign say the chemicals might be dangerous (Hunter, 1971).

Dried fruit gets its share of chemicals. Trays are sprayed with pesticides. "Golden" raisins are bleached, a process which destroys vitamins. Sorbic acid may be added as a preservative. Methyl bromide is used to fumigate dates, dried vegetables, nuts, spices, chocolate and dairy products.

A total raw fruit diet can be dangerous. It can cause mental aberrations such as those caused by alcohol, and also possible heart damage. The fruit probably ferments in the colon and produces more alcohol than the body can handle at one time. It may be that all the sprays on fruit may cause some of the trouble.

To destroy possibly 85 percent of the pesticides on the skin of the fruit, wash it in biodegradable soap and water. Next wash in ¼ cup of distilled vinegar in a dishpanful of water, then rinse in clear water. Canned applesauce often contains more additives than any other fruit.

Let's try to buy all possible dried and fresh fruits and vegetables at a health food store or from nearby farmers who don't ship their produce long distances.

You may want to get fruits in the summer and puree them to make juice in the blender and store it in the freezer. It's easy to make jelly one jar at a time as we need it. It takes only about ten minutes. Recipe p. 102.

In freezing our own, some fruits are really fast and easy. Frozen peaches, strawberries, melons and berries keep well all winter. One of the best ways to use frozen peaches and bananas is in smoothies. They can be made of fresh frozen berries and strawberries, too. These desserts take the place of ice cream.

GELATIN FRUIT TREAT

Whip in blender at high speed:
1 T gelatin from health food store
½ c hot water (from faucet)
Add and blend till smooth, then cool till mixture thickens slightly:
¾ c frozen fruit of any kind
Fill to measure with ice water if fruit is not liquid enough to measure exactly. Add:
2 T lemon juice (optional)
1 c yogurt or milk
1 c fruit in bite-size pieces
2 T honey
½ c cottage cheese
½ c pecans (optional)
Pour into a large, deep pie plate lined with cake slices or with toasted sweetened wheat germ or with cookie crumbs. If you don't have the lining ingredients, serve as is.
Yield: 6–8 servings
Note: This makes eating yogurt easy for those who are reluctant.

FROZEN FRUIT SMOOTHIES

Spread peaches on trays so they don't touch each other, and let them ripen until they're mellow. Then put the trays in the deep freeze until the peaches are frozen hard. Put them in bags and put them back in the freezer. If bagged first, those on the bottom will be mashed by the weight of those on top. They'll keep for a year or more in plastic bags.

One of the best ways to use frozen peaches is to make smoothies. Use one medium frozen peach for each serving. Hold it under the faucet between your hands. Scrub as if you're washing your hands, and the peel will slip right off. Let the peach sit on the counter about two minutes and cut the flesh away from the stone, letting the peach slices drop into the blender. Add about ½ c milk and blend till smooth. You may have to help it along on the top with a rubber spatula. Then add 1 t or so of honey or dark brown sugar. This will be similar to frozen custard—thick enough to eat with a spoon. If you'd rather drink it, just use more milk—about 1 cup per peach. You can make smoothies with any kind of frozen fruit. A friend of mine likes cantaloupe. My favorite is banana, and it doesn't take any honey—the bananas are sweet enough.

To make a banana smoothie, let the bananas ripen till they're mellow. Peel and slice in ½ inch slices. Spread on tray and freeze, then put in plastic bags. They'll keep for one month at zero degrees without turning brown. The rest is the same as the peach, except no sweetening. Strawberries are especially good mixed with banana. They're rather strong flavored if used alone.

If you don't have a zero degree freezer, freeze only enough for one round of smoothies—don't try to store the fruit. Or freeze milk in ice cube pans and use a few milk cubes, a little liquid milk, and cold fruit. If one ingredient is frozen, you'll get the texture of ice cream.

I've served smoothies with a dollop of real whipped cream to many guests. Everybody likes them, even people who are not interested in nutrition but just want something that tastes good.

APPLESAUCE

You can make applesauce easily in the blender. Dice 4 apples. Peel only if waxed. Add a few pieces at a time to blender container with just enough water to get the blender going. Add 1 T lemon juice. Add cinnamon and nutmeg if desired. Eat immediately before it browns.
Yield: 4 servings

PUMPKIN

Wash the kids' Jack O'Lantern (or buy a pumpkin for the purpose) and cut it into squares. Steam it and peel it. Puree in a blender. Use for pumpkin pie, pumpkin bread, or pudding. Freeze in 1 or 2 cup portions, whatever your favorite recipes call for.

JELLIES AND PRESERVES

Freeze purees and juices for raw jellies, gelatins, drinks and punches later in the year. Fill the blender with fruit, add one cup of honey, turn on and off to pull the fruit down, blend till smooth and strain through a medium large wire strainer. Save the peelings and seeds, add water and put in a jar in the fridge. You'll have an extra glass of juice for breakfast (Nusz, 1972). I freeze grape juice this way every year, then use the juice or puree a little at a time and make jelly. The red and dark fruits are best for this. You might like to add 1 tablespoon of apple cider vinegar to two cups or more of grape juice for "wine."

Strawberries are good frozen whole. They must be washed and have the green tip pinched out. Try not to cut the berry; it loses vitamin C. Put the berries upside down on a tray so water won't collect in the cavity. When frozen, place in plastic bags.

Raw jellies are the best kind. Mix 1 cup of the juice or puree with a box of pectin jell. Cook till thick. Add another cup of juice and mix well. In an hour or two, it will be thick. It gets thicker the longer it sets. For a thinner jelly, add more puree. This jelly is half raw fruit which has more food value than cooked. For strawberry preserves, mash some berries for juice. Simmer the juice with pectin for five minutes with ½ cup or so of honey. Add whole fruit and set aside to thicken (Nusz, 1972). Even easier is to boil one cup of honey with a box of pectin. Take off the stove and add chopped whole fruit or puree.

If you ever pick your own figs, here's the easy way to preserve them. Put on trays in the freezer and freeze whole. Wash them when you get them out. When figs are washed, they're hard to dry, and if water stays on them, it freezes; ice crystals seem to make the fruit watery. Bugs can't live at zero degrees anyway. Eat the fruit before it gets quite thawed, or make preserves.

You can make healthful raw fruit preserves with much less sugar than commercial preserves, and have a food that will add flavor and interest to hot cakes, muffins and fruit smoothies all year. You can do this in less time than it takes to read about it.

The little book Frieda Nusz wrote called *The Natural Foods Blender Cookbook* (see References) opened up a new world of quick cookery to me.

FRUIT SYRUPS

Boil and simmer 1 c honey with 1 box apple pectin till thick and glossy. Add a bottle of pure fruit juice or your frozen purees.

Or: Simmer 1 c fruit juice along with the pectin.

Or: For a thicker fruit syrup, use 2 boxes of pectin.

The best syrup is made mostly with raw fruit.

Also: Add whole raw fruits such as blueberries. Any combination seems to be good.

QUICK FRUIT TOPPING

Cook till thick, stirring constantly:
   ½ c juice, such as pineapple
   1 box pectin
Add:
   1½ c frozen fruit
Blend all together. Add sugar if needed. Try frozen strawberries or raspberries.
Yield: about 2 cups

FRUIT FOR DESSERT

Nothing new, but we don't want to forget old favorites. How about a big platter of apple bites (dip them in orange juice so they won't get brown), orange sections, banana chunks, whole dates, pineapple, peach bites, and a few melon balls with pecan halves scattered over all.

CREAMY FRUIT DESSERT

Chill in freezer till crystals form around edges (also chill the egg beater):
  ½ c evaporated milk
Whip milk and add:
  2 T lemon juice (optional)
  4 T honey
  4 T powdered milk
  1 t vanilla or
  ½ t lemon extract
Fold mixture into:
  2 c thick chilled fruit puree—prune, apricot, banana, peach or a combination
Add nuts if desired.
Yield: 6 servings

PEACH OR APRICOT DESSERT

Pour into saucepan to get hot:
  1½ c pineapple or apricot juice
Mix together and stir well:
  ½ c juice (additional)
  2 heaping T cornstarch
Stir cornstarch mixture into hot juice and keep stirring until it is very thick and bubbling.
Add to the hot mixture:
  2 c fresh peaches or fresh or steamed dried apricots in bite-size pieces
  2 egg yolks
  1 t almond extract
Pour into cooked pie crust or serve without crust as pudding.

Variation: Beat egg whites and fold into mixture before chilling.

Or: Make meringue with the two egg whites. Combine and beat with a rotary beater until stiff:
  2 egg whites
  2 T water
  ½ t vanilla
  pinch of salt
Add 2 T at a time:
  ¼ c sugar
Spread meringue over pie and bake at 300 F for 30 minutes.
Yield: 6 servings

CRANBERRY-ORANGE SAUCE

Chop in blender:
  1½ c fresh or frozen cranberries
  1 or 2 organically grown oranges with seeds removed
Add nuts if desired.
Yield: 2 cups

APRICOT GLAZE

Soak overnight:
  ⅓ pound dried apricots (about 2 c)
  1 c water
  ⅓ c sugar
Cook ingredients slowly until the apricots are soft. Blend in blender or processor. Store in fridge or in freezer. To use frozen fruit, let it thaw, dilute it with water and spread it over fruit, cake or pancakes. Or mix with real whipped cream and fill cream puff shells.
Yield: about 4 cups

BANANA FROZEN DESSERT

Here's a nice snack for evening. It has the two ingredients needed for a snack (fruit and protein), so your children may eat and enjoy.

Separate an egg and beat:
  1 egg white
Mix all ingredients together in blender:
  1 egg yolk
  1 peeled apple cut in chunks
  ½ c milk
  1 T non-instant powdered milk
  2 bananas, cut in chunks
  1 T honey or dark brown sugar
Fold in beaten egg white. Pour into a refrigerator tray and freeze about 30 minutes. Beat well and finish freezing.
Yield: 5 servings

FRUIT BUTTER

Wash, core, cut into quarters and cook together slowly until soft:
  2 pounds peaches or apples
  1 c water
Blend in blender. Add and cook until the butter sheets from a spoon:

½ c brown sugar
1 t cinnamon
½ t powdered cloves
¼ t allspice
grated lemon rind and juice (optional)

"Sheeting" is when two large drops form along the edge of the spoon; when the two drops come together, "sheeting" is completed.
Yield: about 3 cups

13

BEVERAGES

IN BRIEF

We don't drink coffee (decaf or real), tea, cola, cocoa, bottled drinks, canned drinks, booze (including beer) or fruit juice.

I know what you're thinking—what's left to drink? Water and milk. Herb tea if you wish (thirty minutes before meals) or a hot drink made from cereal, which you can get at a health food store.

Nut milks are healthful and delicious. Use them on cereal if you like. These milks can also be used as sauce on vegetable roasts.

WATER

Water seems almost like a forgotten drink for adults and for many children who have been brought up on fruit juices or colas in their nursing bottles.

Water is still the best drink, but it can be contaminated. Tap water should be drawn and allowed to stand until the chlorine evaporates out. Anyone can do this; it takes only about an hour. Richard Passwater says he wouldn't give a dog tap water that hadn't been filtered, and he suggests a little filter (under $20) that fits on the sink faucet (Passwater, 1976).

Bottled spring water may or may not be good—some say there are no clean springs in the country. Some former spring water bottling companies are now selling distilled water with minerals added, because the distilled water has no minerals or anything else in it. The minerals already in the tissues of the body can leach out by osmosis if there are no minerals in the water we drink.

Soft water isn't as good to drink as hard water. Soft has more sodium, which most of us don't need. Water softeners aren't good because sodium is used to soften water. Soft water is acid, and it leaches cadmium, a dangerous mineral, from the water pipes. Hard water is alkaline and furnishes minerals, especially calcium, which is helpful to the heart.

When to drink water is important. The first glass of the day should be sitting on your bedside table waiting for you to drink as soon as you wake up. This should be thirty minutes before breakfast. The water will go through the stomach to the intestines, helping peristalis—the muscular movements of the intestine that result in elimination.

We should drink water thirty minutes before each meal and each mid-meal. Drink as much as you're comfortable with, probably 6 to 12 ounces. We're all different. How long after a meal should we drink water? Two hours. Since we eat about every 2½ hours all day, 30 minutes before a meal is the same time on the clock as two hours after.

We drink water before meals so it will go through the stomach into the small intestine before our food gets to the stomach. We need a very acid medium to digest food in the stomach. The hydrochloric acid of the stomach is secreted at a pH of .8, almost as acid as we can measure.

By the time the food we eat mixes with the acid, the pH measures 2 to 3, which is exactly right for our enzymes to digest protein. If we dilute our stomach contents with water or other beverages so it comes up to 4 to 5 on the pH scale, the proteins can't be digested, and they go on through the stomach, twenty feet of small intestine, five feet of large intestine, and stack up in the sigmoid colon—way down in the left side of the body, as undigested, putrified proteins. They cause gas. So much gas is formed that bubbles of gas push up between the muscles in the sigmoid colon, and putrified fecal matter follows. The resulting pouches of skin containing the fecal matter are called diverticula. The ailment is called diverticulosis; or, if the pouches become inflamed, it's called diverticulitis. We have these pouches for life unless they're surgically removed. Diverticulosis is a forerunner of cancer of the colon, the second most common location of cancer in men and women both.

Diverticulosis is also caused by taking antacids, which also dilute the hydrocholoric acid in the stomach. A deficiency of fiber can lead to cancer because without fiber, the fecal matter becomes packed in the intestine and presses against the walls of the colon for long periods of time and causes sore places which may become cancerous.

The undigested proteins can go through the blood vessels in the small intestine, through the liver, and into the main circulation. From there, they can get into the brain or any other cells in the body and cause inflammation. This inflammation shows up as mucus which results in hay fever, skin rash or swelling of tissues in the brain which we can't see, but which causes behavior problems and/or learning disabilities. All these conditions are now called allergies. Of course, we're allergic to foreign invaders in the body, but foreign invaders couldn't get into our cells if the cells were healthy (see *A Home Study Course in the New Nutrition*, Long, 1983).

Many of these problems are caused by drinking water with meals and diluting the hydrocholoric acid. If you forget to drink water thirty minutes before meals, you may need a small amount with meals, otherwise water to mix the food with may be drawn from the tissues, which is bad. But much of the need for water depends on the kinds of food eaten. Muscle meats demand water for processing; fruits and vegetables supply water. Many contain 90 percent or more water—and fruits and vegetables should be a large part of the diet.

Remember, if you're thirsty, regardless of

time, drink. But try to remember to drink water thirty minutes before meals.

SOFT DRINKS

Let's stay away from soft drinks as well as hard. Soft drinks have too much sugar. We can become addicted to sugar in soft drinks, which can help cause fluctuating blood sugar. Low blood sugar (hypoglycemia) can lead to high blood sugar (diabetes, the third-ranking killer disease) if it isn't treated, and the only treatment is diet.

Soft drinks contain many additives, including caffeine. Some cola drinks have caffeine without its being mentioned on the label. Other drinks have caffeine, but the label must say so (Hunter, 1971). The acid and sugar combined in soft drinks can damage tooth enamel. Artificial colors and flavors and one or more of twenty-three allowed preservatives are listed on the label (Goldbeck, 1972).

If soft drinks are artificially sweetened, that's just as bad because of the chemicals, especially phosphates, which in large amounts can destroy calcium in the bones.

Fruit juices have as much sugar as soft drinks. If they're freshly squeezed or pressed, they don't have the other additives that soft drinks have, but they still have sugar. For example, grapefruit juice has five teaspoons of sugar in about seven ounces; orange, four; pineapple, five and one half. All of these have no added sugar; the sugar is what nature put in.

Many of my nutrition students are young mothers who try to feed their children well. They take them off soft drinks and then let them drink apple juice or other fruit juice all day. Some of these children drink eight or ten glasses a day, which adds up to ¾ cup of sugar—natural, but still sugar. That much sugar can cause fluctuations of blood sugar leading to hypoglycemia and then diabetes. Also, fruit juices are often acid and can harm the enamel on the teeth.

Canned or bottled fruit juices are even worse. Some of them are called "drink blend," "ade," "drink," "punch," "nectar," or "flavored drink." These can have as little as 10 percent fruit juice. The rest is water and chemicals, most of which are detrimental to the body.

Canned or bottled vegetable juices are useful as vehicles to mix with desiccated liver or brewer's yeast for better taste. Otherwise, it is usually better to eat the whole raw vegetable.

ALCOHOLIC BEVERAGES

When I speak at club meetings, someone often asks, "You haven't mentioned booze—what about it?" The answer is probably obvious—leave it alone. Many research reports show that animals drink alcohol (when given the choice) only when they're on a poor diet. That tells us that when people are given good nutrition, the craving for alcohol, like that for sugar, will leave.

In fact, if people drink, their nutrition is not as good as it should be because alcohol takes the place of food. Alcohol furnishes only sugar, and many nutritionists say that all alcoholics, without exception, are hypoglycemic (suffering from low blood sugar).

Both alcoholics and sugarholics need good nutrition. "But," you say, "I'm not an alcoholic. I just like my cocktail or two before dinner. I can take it or leave it." Leave it—you'll no doubt feel better. But if you can't leave it, you'll know you're addicted, even if it's to only one or two drinks.

In addition to water without chlorine, what can we drink? Some of the best drinks are whipped up in the blender with nuts, water and pureed fruits. Good nuts to use are almonds, pecans, peanuts, walnuts and Brazil nuts. Almond milk is very alkaline, high in protein and easy to assimilate and absorb. Cantaloupe seed milk is made the same as other nut milks; it must be strained to remove the sharp tips of the seed. Sesame seed milk is good for growing children, for gaining weight and for lubricating the intestines.

NUT MILK

Place in blender and blend till powdery:
    ¼ c chopped nuts
Add slowly and blend until smooth:
    ½ to 1 c water

Flavor with:
    pure vanilla
    carob
    pureed fresh fruit
    dark brown sugar

This is good to drink or to use without flavoring in any recipe that calls for milk.
Yield: ½ to 1 cup

Or: Soak almonds or sunflower seeds overnight in a little water to soften. In blender, blend for 2–3 minutes:
    3 oz. soaked nuts or seeds
    5 oz. water
Flavor as above.

Or: Add peanut butter or any nut butter to a glass of milk.

Or: Use any seeds—sesame, pumpkin, sunflower, watermelon, cantaloupe, muskmelon, ripe cucumber, summer squash, zucchini or any fresh vegetable seeds. Flavor with mint leaves, herbs or dill to taste. Some seeds have sharp points, so strain to remove.

NO-MILK MILK

If anyone is allergic to milk, this makes a good substitute. On this diet, you will soon get over your allergies.

Blend on high speed:
    ½ c sunflower seeds
    3 eggs
    ⅓ c cooked grain—brown rice, oatmeal, or cracked wheat (optional)
    ½ c sesame seeds
    ⅓ c water
Add water to desired consistency. Add fruit or pure vanilla to your taste.
Yield: about 2½ cups

QUICKIE EGG DRINK

When you're in a hurry (this may be every morning) you can drink your egg quickly. This drink is much more healthful than a drink made from protein powders.

In blender:
  1 c whole milk
  1 T lecithin
  1 raw egg
  ¼ to 1 T (or more) brewer's yeast
Flavor with fruit, pure vanilla, almond extract, ½ t dark brown sugar, carob powder or peanut butter.
Yield: 1 or 2 servings

Please note: If you're not used to taking brewer's yeast, it might cause nausea, so begin with ¼ t and build up gradually.

For more protein, add 1 T soy powder (not flour) and/or 1 T non-instant powdered milk. Bran and wheat germ may be added in small amounts if you don't mind the thick texture. You should be putting bran and wheat germ in all your baked goods anyway.

HEALTH DRINK

Have this drink ready for your children when they come home from school. It will keep them from craving junk-food sweets.

Place in a blender and allow to soak for 15 minutes, then blend till smooth:
  ¼ c sunflower seed kernels
  ¼ c sesame seeds
  ½ c cashews or almonds
  3 c cold water
Add and blend till smooth:
  1 to 2 T honey
  pinch of salt to taste
  ½ t soy milk powder
Serve cold.
Yield: 4 to 6 servings

LIVER COCKTAIL

The parents can drink this cocktail. They will never be fatigued or depressed when they drink this high-powered food.

Place in a blender and blend till smooth:
  2 ounces raw calves' liver
    or 1 rounded T desiccated liver
  1 small carrot, quartered
  a pinch of sea salt
  water to the consistency you like
Yield: 1 serving

14

DESSERTS

WHY DESSERTS?

We should all eat as if we were diabetic!

In 70 percent of men who eat the national average of sugar (125 pounds per person per year) the following changes take place: Blood platelets are stickier, thus clots and heart attacks are more common. Blood triglycerides, uric acid and insulin levels rise. Cholesterol deposits increase. The adrenal glands and the liver enlarge. None of these changes is good. Sugar intake causes low blood sugar. Symptoms (there are about 100) range from anxiety to suicidal depression, and from impotence in men to frigidity in women.

Then why do we have a big section on desserts? Because we can eat good, nutritious desserts with small amounts of sugar, say a total of 10-15 pounds a year. And if we all eat as if we were diabetic, we'll never become diabetic.

You'll find many delicious, healthful desserts you can make for your family. If you're so strict that you won't allow any desserts at all, that's up to you, but such strict rules often backfire. As soon as the children go to a neighbor's house to play, they load up on sugar. Or when they get old enough to have their own money, how is anyone going to stop them from spending it on junk food? They should have small amounts of healthful sweets at their own homes.

SUGARS

No sugars are really good. White table sugar is not healthful; neither are brown sugar, raw sugar, turbinado or honey. But a small amount of almost any sugar is not damaging as long as we put plenty of excellent nutrients with it, especially whole grains. Sugar cane itself is healthful; it has many vitamins and minerals. People who chew sugar cane don't get cavities from it. Sugar cane cutters in Africa don't get diabetes. It's just refined sugar that is harmful (Ballentine, 1978). Other names for sugar are dextrose, glucose, molasses, sorbitol and corn sweetener.

Refined sugar is one of the cheapest carbohydrates because it doesn't spoil. It has nothing in it except calories. Foods that spoil need refrigeration and special handling which make them expensive.

DARK BROWN SUGAR: white sugar often sprayed with molasses. But molasses is healthful, so brown sugar is acceptable in small amounts. However, we can never tell if the brown sugar we buy is white sugar mixed with molasses or with syrup made of caramelized white sugar. This product has no trace minerals or anything else but calories.

Make your own dark brown sugar. Buy a 5 pound bag of white sugar. Pour in 1 cup of blackstrap molasses. Stir it in until it's barely moist. You'll be sure you're getting the best brown sugar because blackstrap has vitamins and minerals.

MOLASSES: Molasses is a by-product of refining sugar. Sweet molasses has a fair amount of sugar, but "blackstrap" has less sugar, with lots of iron, some calcium, and plenty of trace minerals such as zinc, copper and chromium. It can also have lead and pesticides (Ballentine, 1978), so we don't use much of it. But since it is an excellent source of minerals, we can use a little.

CORN SWEETENER: Recently, we've been eating much more corn sweetener than ever before, most of it added to foods by manufacturers. Corn syrup is high fructose, which is dangerous in large amounts. The average intake of corn syrup went up from 10.1 pounds per person in 1960 to 32.7 pounds per person in 1976.

HONEY: Many people think it's all right to eat a lot of honey because it doesn't call out the insulin reaction (which may lead to low blood sugar), but there are other reasons for not eating honey. Honey (fructose or levulose) does everything sucrose (white table sugar) does, and does it less desirably. Triglycerides don't begin to clear the blood for nine hours after a high fructose load. With a high sucrose load, the sugar has left the blood by nine hours (Pauling, 1978). Also, our brains feed on glucose, which is half the content of sucrose, but is not found in fructose.

Our energy comes from glucose, and the body must change fructose to glucose in order to use it. We did not evolve using much fructose, and it is thought that the use of fructose has partly caused the high incidence of heart disease.

We shouldn't buy honey that has been cooked or heated. The label should read "raw" or "unheated." Dark brown sugar can be used in recipes that call for cooking. Honey can be added to certain recipes such as sauces after the food is cooked. Cooked honey has an acid off-taste that is very different from raw honey (Ballentine, 1978).

Raw, unstrained honey is best, if we use honey. Clover honey is mildest. Dark, cloudy honey has more vitamins and minerals than clear honey. If honey crystallizes, put it in an oven on low heat. That's better than putting the jar in a pan of warm water on the stove because the bottom would get hotter than the rest. Honey keeps well indefinitely. The main advantage of eating honey is that it is sweeter than white sugar, and it takes less to sweeten foods.

SORGHUM AND CANE SYRUP: Good foods. They are juices with only water removed, but pure cane syrup doesn't keep very long, so it isn't usually available. Genuine raw sugar is natural sugar cane juice which is dried and ground. But it isn't available because the law says sugar must be purified (Ballentine, 1978).

TURBINADO: Raw sugar. It is so contaminated by soil, molds, yeasts and bacteria that it has to be washed with steam, so it isn't very different from white sugar. It may have traces of chromium (Ballentine, 1978), but not enough to help.

DATE SUGAR: Made from ground dried dates. It's good for fruit-crisp toppings. It doesn't dissolve as white sugar does, but it makes good cookies and muffins.

PURE MAPLE SYRUP: Has more food value than some of the other sweeteners. Rather than using one tablespoon of white sugar, which has only 0.6 mg calcium, 0.01 mg iron, 0.1 mg phosphorus and a trace of potassium and copper, we may use one tablespoon of pure maple syrup, which has 21 mg calcium, 0.24 mg iron, 1.6 mg phosphorus and 35 mg potassium. Real maple syrup will sweeten cookies, pies, cakes and other desserts which are made with whole grains, real butter, yard eggs and whole milk, fortified with soy powder and non-instant powdered milk, and made more appetizing and more healthful with plenty of nuts and seeds.

We may use carob, maple sugar and many fruits as sweeteners. When we use health food cookbooks, let's use half the amount of sugar the recipe calls for. You can start with more, if your family insists, but try to reduce the amount to half as soon as possible. When we eat less sugar, our tastes change, and the old too-sweet foods we used to eat become repulsive to our tastes.

SYNTHETIC SWEETENERS

The synthetic sweetener saccharin is still allowed on the market, although tests show that it causes tumors in animals. This was reported in 1951 by Food and Drug Administration scientists, but the report was ignored. Dozens of articles have been published showing the dangers of saccharin. Dr. George T. Bryan, a tumor expert and cancer researcher, reported that 52 percent of the animals in one experimental group taking saccharin got bladder cancer. He commented that saccharin should be used only by those who have a medical reason for using it, and that "it may be many years before it is known exactly how dangerous the substance is."

Saccharin, is a noxious drug and is harmful to the human system even in small doses, according to Dr. Harvey W. Wiley (1913). Dr. Wiley was responsible for much good legislation in the food industry. France banned saccharin in 1890, and other countries followed suit. As early as 1951, FDA scientists reported that saccharin may cause cancer, but nothing was done (Hunter, 1971).

Cyclamates were developed in 1950, but they were supposed to be used carefully only by certain individuals, not by the general public. Reports from investigators show that cyclamates can cause death of a fetus, diarrhea, weight gain and growth retardation. They cause diseases of the kidney, liver, intestinal tract, adrenal glands and thyroid glands, bring about adverse reactions with other drugs such as antibiotics and anticoagulants and even cause chromosome breakage which could result in genetic damage. Cyclamates were finally removed from the market.

NATURAL SWEETENERS

What kind of sugar should we eat? Best is to sweeten with fruits, fresh or dried—raisins, dates, apricots, etc. Or use small amounts of molasses, dark brown sugar, maple syrup or sorghum molasses.

The best idea is to eat less sugar, or none, until your tastes change. Before long, sweets will taste too sweet, and very small amounts of sugar or other sweeteners will be enough.

When I had been on my "new" health food diet for several months, every once in a while someone would ask me, "Don't you ever want to eat something that tastes good?" Many people believe that natural food enthusiasts, or "health fooders," as I call myself, never get to eat any desserts or foods that are sweet. "Good" seems to be exactly related to sweets in most people's minds.

I would always say, "Everything I eat tastes good, or I wouldn't eat it." But to be specific, health fooders can eat sweets. It's just that we're very choosy about the amount of sugar and the kinds of sweeteners we use, as well as what else we eat with the sweets.

In the first place, most of us get over our craving for sugar. It might not be easy for everyone, but it was for me. I had been a coffee-sugarholic, with some kind of sweet and coffee every two to three hours all day. When I changed my diet, I stopped sweets cold turkey, in one day; but I tapered off coffee to avoid the withdrawal headaches. Within a few days I felt so much better that I wouldn't have gone back to my old ways for the sake of any candy bar or piece of pie.

Finally, after several months, I wanted a certain kind of candy bar. I used to be so crazy about them that my husband often gave me one for Christmas. But when I took the first bite, I had to spit it out—it was so sweet that it was repulsive to my taste.

I still like natural sweets, and always have cookies, candy or some dessert on hand in the freezer. But every dessert I eat builds health and tastes better than the old super-sweet desserts I used to like. Part of the fun of this natural food regimen has been collecting recipes for and making new desserts, because we must make our own.

FRUITS

Fruits, of course, are obviously healthful sweets. The kids might not go for them at first. Maybe we can make them rather special. A fruit plate to be passed around might be appealing. Fruit cups and whips with or without real whipped cream are special.

With a meal of a hearty soup or salad, serve a high-protein dessert, such as a baked custard, cheesecake or nut torte. Combinations of ground nuts, seeds, honey and eggs make delicious tortes, served plain or with a fruit glaze. Cheese-cake is good made with cottage cheese (high in protein) rather than with cream cheese (high in fat). Serve your dessert at the next snack time rather than with the meal. An important rule of good nutrition is to never overeat.

Other proteins to add to desserts are soy powder, peanut flour, nuts, seeds and eggs. Add or substitute for part of the flour: Brazil nuts, sunflower seeds, almonds or soy grits. We make all kinds of cakes, candy, cookies, ice cream, custards, pie, puddings with extra powdered milk for protein and calcium, extra wheat germ for B vitamins and protein, and soy powder and eggs for many nutrients.

COOKIES AND CAKES

You would probably never feed a store-bought cookie to your family if you realized that it is made with white sugar, white flour, imitation eggs with egg color from nitric acid, chemical improvers, "mineral oil pan grease," "cultured butter flavor" which is advertised to add "that special touch of richness which tastes exactly like butter in finished goods—It needs no refrigeration—guaranteed to stay sweet and fresh; a single ounce will flavor 60 pounds of dough"; artificial dyes, caramel coloring, flavor enhancers and cheap imitation flavors. Peanut flavoring can be made without peanuts. Hundreds of artificial flavors are on the shelves at spice and flavoring manufacturing plants. Their reason for being is their low cost and their ability to stay fresh, it seems, practically forever.

Here are cookies we can eat. They're made with whole grain flour and/or nut flour—maybe a combination of two or three that furnish different nutrients (try ⅓ wholewheat flour, ⅓ soy, and ⅓ wheat germ for a tasty combination), fresh yard eggs, fresh whole milk, fresh flavorings and pure vanilla. Use wheat germ, ground or whole seeds, chopped nuts, soy powder and powdered milk for extra protein, vitamins and minerals; and for the little sweetening our new taste requires, chopped dates, raisins or date sugar, all of which have vitamins and minerals along with their sweetness, or a little dark brown sugar which has small amounts of vita-mins and minerals. Every bite of such desserts builds health.

I don't often use my old favorite recipes; I'd rather use new natural food recipes, but there's one I like. It's angel food cake. I accumulate a lot of egg whites because we sometimes use raw egg yolks in sauces. When we have 1¼ cups of whites, I make an angel food cake. I just substitute dark brown sugar or honey for white sugar (half as much as the recipe calls for), and I substitute wholewheat flour for white. Everybody I've served that cake to likes it, whether he's interested in good nutrition or not, because the cake tastes so good. It rises about half as high as with white flour and sugar, but the flavor is delightful and the texture is moist. See p. 115 for recipe.

PIES

Health food pies are so good you'll wonder how you ever ate the other kind. The crusts, which you probably never ate on ordinary pies because they were like soggy cardboard, are crisp and delicious and so varied you'll have fun trying new ones. To start with the usual ingredients, it's best to chill the butter, cut it into the flour till the pieces are the size of large peas, use ice water, and have the oven temperature high so the pieces of butter will stay separate. This makes a flaky crust. If you use melted butter or warm ingredients, you'll get a delicious crisp crust, but not a flaky one. The easiest way to combine ingredients is in a processor. It's nice to add wheat germ, rice polish, soy flour or powdered milk for extra nutrients. Crumb crusts do well. If you ever have any crackers, cookies, cake or granola that didn't get eaten, blend in the processor or blender to crumbs. Recipes follow.

There is only one sensible way (I think) to get pie crusts into the pan. That's to pat them in. Just mix all ingredients, and instead of rolling them out with a rolling pin on a board—too time-consuming—pat them into the pan with your fingers. Pat dough up the sides, as evenly as you can. It doesn't take long. Then if you have another pie pan just a shade smaller, press the smaller pan on the dough, give it a few quick twists, and you have a nice smooth crust. Of course, you really don't need the crusts. Any pie filling will make a good pudding.

GELATIN DESSERTS

Commercial gelatin desserts have been eaten for years, but they shouldn't have been. They are full of sugar and are greatly unbalanced in amino acids. We can eat them if we use less sugar and add protein—milk or cottage cheese and nuts—for a better amino acid balance. We use gelatin from the health food store.

CAROB

Anybody with a yen for chocolate can have something that tastes the same but, unlike chocolate, builds health. It's carob. It's a naturally sweet, high-complex carbohydrate, with plenty of B vitamins and minerals. It has half the calories of chocolate, 1/100 the amount of fat, and two and a half times as much calcium (Gerras, 1972). Carob comes in powder form like cocoa, in chips and in chunks. Three level tablespoons of carob powder plus two tablespoons liquid equals one square of chocolate.

Carob is good when added to hot cakes or waffles (serve these with real whipped cream or homemade whipped topping), cakes, cookies, smoothies, puddings, candies, icings and even yogurt. Add a little grated orange rind to cakes made with carob. Even add ½ teaspoon of carob to your breakfast yeast drink. I even add one teaspoon to my banana smoothie. Make fudgsicles for the kids—any age. A carob cornstarch pudding works well in fudgsicle forms. Carob has a kind of raw taste. If this bothers your family, dissolve the carob in hot water or in a little melted butter before mixing it with the water. I made a carob sauce once that got grainy when it was cooked. Just a few minutes in the blender made it smooth.

CANDY

We can even eat candy—health food, slightly sweet candy. Start with nuts and seed butters, peanut, sesame, sunflower and almond, all eas-ily made in the blender. Combine with coconut, carob, honey, soy powder, chopped nuts, seeds or dried fruits in your favorite combinations. If you need more liquid, use milk or water. Form into balls, roll in coconut, carob or ground nuts.

WHIPPED TOPPINGS

These are super for any kind of dessert, and we can make them so they build health. One way to make desserts taste sweeter is to chew them a long time. Starch turns to sugar in the mouth. Starch is the best kind of carbohydrate because it allows our blood sugar to go up slowly and stay level, not too high and not too low. Starches furnish energy for many hours.

PASTRY

In making pastry with wholewheat flour and butter, use ice cold water or milk and water, or just milk. Grated cheese, herbs, spices or ground nuts and/or coconut may be mixed with the dry ingredients. The dough can be refrigerated for up to two days or frozen for up to three months. Let it come to room temperature before patting it into pans. An 8-inch pan takes 1½ cups of flour for a 2-crust pie.

BASIC METHOD PIE CRUST

Combine and mix well:
  1½ c wholewheat flour
  1 c wheat germ
  ½ t salt
Add and mix with pastry blender to coarse meal:
  ½ c cold butter (1 stick)
Add and mix well:
  ⅓ c cold water
  Press into pie pan. Fill with uncooked filling and bake 8 minutes at 425 F, lower heat and finish cooking at 325 F.
Or: Bake crust for 8 minutes, fill with uncooked filling and bake at 325 F for 40-50 minutes.
Yield: Enough for 1 8″ or 9″ 2-crust pie or 2 8″ one-crust pies

BASIC METHOD FOR PROCESSOR

Combine and process (steel blade):
   1½ c wholewheat flour
   1 c wheat germ
   ½ t salt
Add and process to coarse meal:
   ½ c cold butter cut in chunks
Pour in chute and process to sticky crumbs:
   ⅓ c cold water
Pat into two 8″ pie pans (see p. 113). Cook as above.
Yield: 2 8″ shells

SOFT BUTTER PASTRY

Pastry made with soft butter is easier made this way:
In bowl, mix with fork:
   5 T soft butter
   2 T cold water
   ½ c wholewheat flour
Add:
   1 c flour
   ¼ t salt
Chill, pat into 8-inch pan, and cook about 16 minutes at 350 F. Fill and finish cooking.
Yield: 1 8″ shell

SWEET PASTRY

In bowl, mix with fork:
   1½ c wholewheat or oat flour
   2 T dark brown sugar
   ¼ t salt
   5 T soft butter
   1 egg yolk beaten with
   1 T cold water
Mix and bake as in basic method.
Yield: 1 9″ pie shell

EASIEST PIE CRUST

Have you tried this one? One-half cup each of wheat germ, shredded coconut and ground pecans mixed and pressed into a pie plate? Easy and quick.

SPECIAL NUT PIE CRUST

Use basic method or basic processor method.

Blend to powder:
   ⅓ c almonds
Add and mix well:
   1½ c whole grain oat or wheat flour
Add and mix to coarse meal:
   6 T butter
Add and mix to sticky crumbs:
   4–6 T cold water
Press dough into pie pan (see p. 113), and bake as in basic method.
Yield: 1 9″ shell

CHEESE PIE CRUST OR CHEESE STRAWS

Mix well:
   ¾ c wholewheat flour
   ¼ t dry mustard (optional)
   ¼ t salt
   ½ c finely grated sharp cheese
Add and mix well:
   ¼ to ½ c water
Pat dough into pan. Fill and bake.

Good with fruit pies, main-dish vegetable pies, even cheese pies.
Yield: 1 8″ shell

Or: Pat dough on a cookie sheet lined with foil until the dough is ¼ inch thick. Score into "straws." Cook at 350 F about eight minutes. Or use the same method used in making Jump-On Crackers, p. 79.
Yield: about 12 straws

GRANOLA PIE CRUST

Blend in blender ½ c at a time, to a fine meal:
   2 c granola
Add and mix well:
   ½ c wheat germ
   1 T non-instant powdered milk
Pour over dry ingredients and mix well:
   ¼ c melted butter
Press into pie pan or spring mold and fill with cheesecake (see p. 116).
Yield: 2 8″ crusts

PIE FILLINGS

PUMPKIN PIE FILLING

Place all ingredients in blender and blend till smooth:
    2 eggs
    ½ c dark brown sugar
    1 t cinnamon
    ⅛ t ground cloves
    ½ c whole milk
    1¾ c pumpkin pulp
    ½ t sea salt
    ½ t ground ginger
    1 c evaporated milk
Pour into a prepared pie shell or buttered pudding pan and bake about 8 minutes at 425 F; reduce heat to 350 F and bake 45 minutes longer.
Yield: 8 servings

FRUIT PIES

Mix together thoroughly:
    ½ c dark brown sugar
    2–3 T wholewheat pastry flour
    pinch of salt
Add:
    3-4 cup fruit in large chunks
Spread filling over prepared pie shell. Top crust is not needed. If crust is not baked, bake at 425 F for 8 minutes; lower heat to 325 F and continue baking 30-35 minutes. If crust is baked, bake at 325 F for 35-45 minutes.
Yield: 6 servings

AMAZING COCONUT PIE

Set oven at 350 F. Combine in blender and blend on low for 3 minutes:
    4 eggs
    ½ c wholewheat flour
    1 t vanilla
    2 c milk
    ½ stick melted butter
Pour into 1 lightly greased 9-inch pan. Let rest for 5 minutes. Sprinkle on custard and press in till moist:
    1 c fresh coconut or one 7-oz. can coconut
Bake for 30 minutes. The crust will be on the bottom.
Yield: 6 servings

PUDDING PIE

Mix well in blender:
    ⅓ to ½ c honey
    ¼ c wholewheat pastry flour
    2 c fresh milk
    ½ c powdered milk
    pinch of salt
    2 egg yolks
Cook, stirring constantly for eight minutes, and add:
    1 T butter
    1 t vanilla
Bake in 8-inch crumb crust or baked shell about 35–40 minutes at 325 F.

Variation: Pour over sweetened fruit in pie crust and bake.
Yield: 6 servings

CAKES

ANGEL FOOD CAKE

This is my old favorite recipe that I've changed to the new flour and sugar. It's about half as tall as when made the old way (with white sugar and flour) but everyone I've served this cake to likes it. It's moist and has a delicious flavor.

Beat in large bowl of electric mixer at high speed till frothy (about 1 minute):
    1¼ c egg whites (about 10 whites)
    ½ t salt
Add and beat three minutes:
    1 t cream of tartar
Add:
    2 T water
Continue beating at high speed till whites will stand in peaks, about 3–4 minutes. Turn mixer to low and add gradually:
    1 c dark brown sugar or ¾ c honey
    ½ t vanilla
    ½ t almond extract
Beat about ½ minute longer. Fluff in bag (do not sift) and fold in by hand:
    ¾ c wholewheat flour
Pour batter into ungreased angel food pan. Bake

about 45 minutes at 325 F. When done, invert and cool 1½ hours.
Yield: 12 servings

CHEESECAKE

Spread an 8×8×2″ pan with butter. Sprinkle with one or a combination of these crumbs, pat down and set aside:
    wholewheat bread crumbs
    coconut
    wheat germ
    ground pecans
Combine in blender in order and whirl:
    2 eggs
    2 t vanilla
    ½ c honey
    2 c cottage cheese
    ¾ t almond extract
    ¼ c powdered milk
Pour filling into crust. Set pan on rack or on jar tops in pan of water. Bake at 300 F for about 45 minutes.
Yield: 8 servings

GINGERBREAD

Preheat oven to 350 F. Grease and flour a 9½″ springform pan (or other similar size). Cream well:
    ½ c soft butter
    ¼ c warmed honey
Add and beat well:
    1 c molasses
    2 t powdered ginger
    1 t nutmeg
    ½ c warm milk
    1 t cinnamon
    ⅓ c brandy (optional)
Beat well and add alternately:
    3 eggs
    2 ⅞ c wholewheat pastry flour combined with
        1 t cream of tartar
Stir in:
    juice of 1 large orange (⅓ cup)
    1 T grated orange rind
Combine and add:
    1 t soda
    1 T warm water
Add and stir well:
    1 c seeded raisins

Bake about 1 hour or till top feels firm.
Yield: 12 servings

BLENDER CAKE

Combine in bowl and mix well:
    ¼ c wheat germ
    1 c wholewheat flour
    ¼ t sea salt
    ⅓ c non-instant powdered milk
    3 T carob (sifted)
    1½ t baking powder
Combine in blender and mix well:
    ⅓ c butter cut in small chunks
    1 c hot water from faucet
    1 t vanilla
    ½ c dark brown sugar
Combine mixtures; pour into 8 or 9″ square pan. Bake at 350 F, 25 minutes.

This is a simple cake with a good flavor. You may add whatever your family likes: carob chips, coconut, nuts, raisins, etc.
Yield: 9 servings

OATMEAL RAISIN CAKE

Set oven at 350 F. Scald:
    1 c milk
Mix with:
    ¼ c butter
    1 c raw oat flakes
    ¼ c honey or dark brown sugar
Cool and add:
    1 egg
In large bowl, mix:
    1½ c wholewheat pastry flour
    2 t cinnamon
    4 t baking powder
Pour liquids into dries, mix, then add:
    ½ c raisins
Pour into 8×8×2″ pan and bake 25–30 minutes.

Glaze
Combine and spread over cake:
    ½ c honey
    ¼ c walnuts chopped
    ¼ c grated coconut
    ½ t vanilla
    1 t butter

Place under broiler 3–4 minutes.
Yield: 10 servings

FRUIT UPSIDE DOWN CAKE

Set oven at 350 F. Combine and bring to boil, stirring constantly, then cool and set aside:
 ¾ c honey or dark brown sugar
 1 c hot water
Combine in bowl and mix well:
 1 c wholewheat flour
 ½ c chopped nuts
 1½ t baking powder
 ½ t salt
 ½ c dark brown sugar or honey
In blender:
 ½ c milk
 2 T butter
 2 eggs
 1 t vanilla
Pour blender mix over dry ingredients and mix well. Pour into 9″ square pan. Add to sugar/water mixture:
 1 c any fresh fruit or organically grown dried fruit
Pour fruit sauce over cake. Bake for 30 minutes. The fruit will be on the bottom when cooked.
Yield: 9 servings

DATE-NUT LOAF

One of the best, yet simple and easy. I always make this at Christmas time.

Mix well:
 ¾ c wholewheat flour
 ½ t salt
 ¼ c wheat germ
 ½ c powdered milk
Sprinkle the flour mixture over:
 1 pound dates, pitted and chopped
Mix till dates are well coated. Blend in blender and combine with date mixture:
 ½ c honey
 1 t pure vanilla
 ½ c soft butter
 3 T grated orange rind
Add:
 1 pound nuts, coarsely chopped
Fold in:
 4 egg whites, stiffly beaten

Turn into oiled and floured 9×5″ loaf pan lined with paper. Bake at 350 F for one hour.
Yield: 18 servings

HOT FUDGE PUDDING CAKE

Set oven at 350 F. Mix well:
 1 c wholewheat flour
 2 t baking powder
 ¼ t salt
 ½ c dark brown sugar or honey
 2 T carob powder
Add and stir well:
 ½ c milk
 2 T butter
  melted in pan you'll bake in
Blend in:
 1 c chopped nuts
Spread in a 9″ square pan. Sprinkle with mixture of:
 ½ c brown sugar (packed)
 ¼ c carob
Pour over entire batter and bake 45 minutes:
 1¾ c hot water
Yield: 9 servings

During baking, cake mixture rises to top and carob sauce sinks to bottom. Serve warm if you wish, with homemade ice cream.

RICH CAROB CAKE

Combine in bowl and mix well:
 2 c wholewheat pastry flour
 ½ c carob, sifted
Combine in blender and buzz:
 6 egg yolks
 ½ c honey
 2 t vanilla
 ⅓ c soft butter
 ⅓ c water
 ½ t salt
Pour liquids over solids and mix well.
Fold in:
 6 egg whites, stiffly beaten
Bake in 9″ springform pan. Bake about 45 minutes at 350 F. Or bake in two 9″ cake pans about 30 minutes at 350 F.
Yield: 12 servings

EASY-ICED CAKE

Please try this cake. It really is easy and good.

Combine in blender and whirl:
¼ c milk
½ c honey
1 t vanilla
¼ c butter melted in pan you'll bake in
3 eggs
Reserve ½ c of this mixture for icing. Combine in bowl and mix well:
½ c unsifted soy powder
¼ c powdered milk
½ t salt
½ c wheat germ
2 t baking powder
Pour remaining liquids over solids and mix well. Pour into 9 × 9 × 1″ pan.

Return the reserved ½ c of liquid mix to blender. Add and blend:
2 T carob powder
Pour over cake batter in a crisscross design. Sprinkle on top:
½ c broken nut meats
Bake at 350 F for 30 minutes.

Note: This batter should be thin enough so icing goes "in." It makes chocolatey lumps with nuts all through the cake.
Yield: 9 servings

SPICY CARROT CAKE

Set oven at 300 F. In saucepan, boil 10 minutes and let cool:
1½ c grated carrots
1½ c raisins
1½ t allspice
¾ t nutmeg
3 T butter
¾ c brown sugar
1½ t cinnamon
1½ t salt
¼ t powdered cloves
Mix well in large bowl:
2¼ c wholewheat pastry flour
1½ t baking soda
¾ c wheat germ
¾ c chopped walnuts or pecans

Pour liquids into dries, mix well and turn into 2 small loaf pans or a ring mold. Bake 45 minutes.
Yield: 12 servings

FROSTING

Blend all ingredients in blender till smooth:
2 T butter
¼ c honey
1 t vanilla
⅔ c non-instant powdered milk
4 T cream
Spread on warm cake.

Or: Add 2 T carob powder in place of 2 T milk powder.
Yield: enough for an 8- or 9-inch square cake.

COOKIES

When we make good cookies, they can be very healthful. We use non-instant powdered milk, wheat germ, soy flour, soy grits, nuts, seeds (powdered if you wish), whole eggs, whole milk, real butter and, as sweeteners, small amounts of raisins, dates, date sugar, honey, dark brown sugar, maple syrup or molasses.

Cookies made with soy or powdered milk may burn more easily. Cook at 25 degrees lower temperature.

OATMEAL COOKIES

Preheat oven to 375 F. Mix in processor (steel blade):
1 c wholewheat pastry flour
(or bread flour)
1 c wheat germ
1 t salt
1½ t baking powder
1 c brown sugar
Add and mix well:
½ c (1 stick) butter cut in
small (¼ inch) pieces
Empty into large bowl and add:
3 c rolled oats
½ package carob chips or raisins
1 c pecans, chopped.
Mix well with fork in 2–cup measure:

2 eggs
3 t vanilla
milk, to total 1¼ c liquid
Add to dry ingredients, mix well, drop on cookie sheet, bake about 12 minutes.
Yield: 6 dozen cookies

CAROB CHEWS

Preheat oven to 350 F. Beat together till light:
2 eggs
⅓ c honey
Stir in the following:
5 T wholewheat flour
1 c chopped nuts
½ c sesame seeds
2 T carob powder
¼ t sea salt
Spread in a buttered 9″ square pan. Cook about 15 minutes. Cool in pan. Cut into squares. When cool, refrigerate or freeze.
Yield: 16 cookies

PROBLY-THE-BEST BROWNIES

Preheat oven to 325 F. In blender:
½ c dark brown sugar
2 eggs
½ c soft butter
½ t vanilla
In bowl:
½ c wholewheat flour
1 t baking powder
3 T carob powder
½ c soy powder or flour
½ t sea salt
Pour liquids over the dries. Mix well, pour into a buttered 9″ square pan. Bake 20–25 minutes. Cut into squares while still slightly warm. Freeze or refrigerate.
Yield: 2 dozen cookies

NUT AND FRUIT BRITTLE

Chop in blender or processor:
1 c dates
1 raw egg
Combine in bowl with:
1 c whole nut meats
2 T wheat germ

Mix well, spread in buttered pan. Bake about ½ hour at 350 F. Break into pieces.
Yield: 2 dozen cookies

SESAME CHEWS

Blend in bowl:
1 c sesame seeds
½ t vanilla
⅓ c honey
Add to stiffen:
soy powder
or non-instant powdered milk
Spread in buttered 8-inch square pan and let harden. Chill. The squares will be dry and are eaten like cookies.
Yield: 16 cookies

SESAME NIBBLES
Mix well and roll into balls:
1 c tahini or powdered sesame seeds
¼ c chopped nuts
3 T wheat germ
¼ c maple syrup or 2 T honey
2 T coconut
4 T carob powder
2 t vanilla
Coat with toasted sesame seeds or coconut. Store in fridge.
Yield: 2 dozen balls

FRUIT NUT STICKS

Combine in blender and whirl till nuts and fruit are chopped in coarse pieces:
2 c nuts
2 eggs
1 c dates or prunes pitted, or dried apricots lightly steamed
Add and make a stiff dough:
¾ c wholewheat flour
¼ c wheat germ
Pat into a 9×9×1″ pan. Bake at 375 F for 15 minutes.
Yield: 20 sticks

TRAVEL OR SNACK BARS

Combine in bowl and mix well:
2 c granola
or 1 c wholewheat bread crumbs and 1 c wheat germ

(or part bran with either choice of ingredients)
    ¼ t salt
    1 c carob chips
    1 t vanilla
    ¾ c wholewheat flour
    ¾ c sesame seeds
Combine in blender and whirl:
    1 egg
    ¼ c honey
    ½ c soft butter
    2 T milk
Pour blender mix into bowl mix. Stir well. Pat the dough into a buttered 9 × 9 × 1″ pan. Bake at 375 F for 15–20 minutes. Cut in oblongs, Easy to carry in purse or brief case for a mid-meal snack or when traveling.

Variation: Drop by spoonfuls on cookie sheet. Substitute chopped pecans for sesame seeds if you wish.
Yield: 20 bars

CREAMY DESSERTS

CAROB CUSTARD

Combine in blender in order given:
    1 c milk
    2 T carob powder
    3 heaping T soy powder
    3 more cups milk
Heat till almost boiling and add:
    3 eggs beaten with
    1 T cornstarch or arrowroot
Cook, stirring constantly till thick. Remove from heat and add:
    1 t pure vanilla
Top with chopped nuts if desired.
Yield: 6 servings

Note: This recipe makes good frozen ice bars.

BAVARIAN CREAM

Pour 1 c canned evaporated milk into small bowl. Freeze till crystals form around edges.

Soak:
    1 T gelatin in 2 T cold water
Scald and mix with softened gelatin:

    1 c milk
    ¼ c carob powder (optional)
Add and chill till thick, not set:
    ⅓ c dark brown sugar or honey
    1½ t vanilla
    ¼ t sea salt
    ¼ t almond extract (optional)
Add and fold in the whipped evaporated milk.
Chill until set.
Yield: 6 servings

CREAM PUFF SHELLS

Cream puffs are easy and fun to make. They freeze well, but they take up a lot of room in the freezer.

Heat in a small saucepan:
    ½ c water
    ¼ c butter
Add all at once:
    ⅜ c wholewheat flour
    ⅛ t salt
Cook and stir until mixture leaves side of pan.
Add one at a time and stir:
    2 unbeaten eggs
Place spoons of batter in 2″ rounds on greased cookie sheet. Bake at 400 F for ½ hour. Reduce heat to 350 F for 5 minutes. Remove from oven, cool and fill with custard or meat dish.
Yield: 16 shells

SUPER SPECIAL PARTY DESSERT

This will be easy if you make it in stages. Make the cake first and freeze it.

Make angel food cake (p. 115). Cool; slice in ½″ slices. Butter two pans, line with sliced cake—bottom and sides.

Slice any fresh or home frozen fruit, one or a combination. I've used strawberries alone and combined with peaches, fresh pineapple and bananas. Heat fresh pineapple to destroy enzymes—you'll be adding gelatin later, and it won't set if you use uncooked pineapple. Pour 3 T kirsch or cherry vodka and 3 T brown or white sugar or honey over the fruit, and mix well. Pour fruit over the cake in pan.

Next make Bavarian cream. Put 1 c canned evaporated milk in a bowl in the freezer till ice crystals form around edges. Soak 1 T health food store gelatin in 2 T water till soft. Add to 1 c scalded milk. Stir till dissolved. In blender, beat 4 egg yolks with ⅓ c sugar or honey till light. Add egg yolk mixture to milk and gelatin. Cool. Whip the evaporated milk, then add 3 T cherry brandy to the egg mix, and fold in the 1 c milk whipped till soft peaks form. Pour over fruit; chill till set.

Variations: Blend ¼ c carob powder with hot milk after gelatin is dissolved.
Yield: 12 servings

QUICKIE RICE PUDDING

Mix 1 c leftover brown rice with ⅓ c yogurt, 2 T raisins and 2 T chopped nuts. A little dark brown sugar is all right if you insist.
Yield: 2 servings

RAISIN BREAD PUDDING

A friend I've known since the early days of my nutrition career keeps me posted with unusually good recipes. Here's one she gave me.

Set oven at 350 F. Soak in hot water 15 minutes:
   ½ c raisins
Cut into cubes and arrange in bottom of a 10 × 6 × 2″ baking dish:
   5 or 6 slices of day-old bread, buttered (obviously this will be homemade whole grain bread)
Sprinkle raisins on top of bread. Mix well and pour over bread:
   3 beaten eggs
   ¼ t salt
   ⅓ c brown sugar, packed
   3 c milk
   1 t vanilla (optional)
Let soak 10 minutes, sprinkle cinnamon over top, and bake 25–30 minutes.
Yield: 12 servings

GELATIN DESSERTS

Packaged gelatin desserts are 85 percent sugar, and the proteins are out of balance. Here's an easy way to avoid both situations.

Sprinkle 1 T of health food store gelatin over ½ c of cold fruit in a saucepan to soften. When soft, place the saucepan over low heat and stir till the gelatin dissolves—2–3 minutes. Remove from heat; add 1¼ c more pureed fruit and 2–4 T honey. Pour mix into bowl and chill.

Now to add protein: add chopped nuts, ground seeds, cottage cheese; also fruit if you wish.

Variation: Let the mixture chill till slightly thick, and beat with an electric or rotary beater till frothy. Chill and add any of above proteins or fruits. Or chill the original mix till slightly thick; fold in one cup evaporated milk or cream whipped. Or fold in fruit and nuts before adding cream. The "whipped cream" may be a whipped topping from this book.
Yield: about 6 servings

ICE CREAM

To make ice cream in the electric ice cream freezer, the Champion juicer or the blender or food processor,

scald:
   6 c milk
In blender, blend:
   2 c milk
   1 c honey
   12 eggs
Add to scalded milk, cook at low heat, stirring constantly until mixture coats spoon. I stir with a rubber spatula in one hand, spoon in the other. Dip the spoon frequently, and you won't over-cook. Cook and add:
   1 T vanilla
Pour into freezer can. Fill with additional whole milk till mix is two inches from top of can. Freeze.

For Champion juicer:
Freeze in large flat pan (9 × 12″ cake pan is good). Cut in strips and put through feeding tube of juicer. Be sure to chill the parts of the juicer that will touch the frozen custard.

For blender:
Freeze in large flat pan. Cut in chunks, blend

quickly and refreeze. Or blend chunks with frozen fruit of your choice.
Yield: 12 servings

CAROB-BANANA ICE CREAM/PUDDING

Process (plastic blade) till smooth:
    3–4 ripe bananas
    3 T carob powder
    ¼ c tahini
    ¼ c natural peanut butter
    2 T chopped pecans
Spoon into four small dessert dishes. Sprinkle with coconut if desired. Cover with foil. Refrigerate for use as pudding or freeze for "ice cream."
Yield: 4 servings

FRUIT SHERBET

Freeze 1 c fruit puree slowly to a soft mush. Fold in ½ c whipped evaporated milk. Add a little honey if needed. Finish freezing.
Yield: 4 servings

CHOCOLATE MOUSSE

Pour into bowl and freeze till ice crystals form around edge:
    1 large can evaporated milk
Sprinkle gelatin on top of water and set aside until soft:
    1½ t gelatin
    2 T cold water
Heat in a saucepan or top of double boiler (do not boil):
    1 c carob chips
    1 c milk
    ⅜ c dark brown sugar
        or ¼ c honey
Pour into mixing bowl and beat with rotary beater. Add:
    1 t vanilla
Add gelatin and mix till melted. Chill till thick then beat with rotary beater till light and fluffy. Whip the evaporated milk until stiff and fold into chocolate mixture.

Return mousse to freezer until time to serve.
Yield: 6–8 servings

TOPPINGS AND SAUCES

VANILLA DESSERT TOPPING

This is a delightful, healthful topping, non-fattening, easy to make, but it takes 10 minutes mixing time. Don't try to make it in a blender—it won't work.

Beat with electric mixer till soft peaks form, about 5 minutes:
    ½ c ice water
    ½ c non-instant powdered milk
Add and beat five more minutes:
    1 t vanilla
    2 T honey
Refrigerate and use within two hours.
Yield: 1 cup

WHIPPED TOPPING

Blend in blender:
    1 t gelatin
    2 t cold water
Add and beat:
    3 T boiling water
Add and beat:
    ½ c ice water
    3 T sugar or 2 T honey
    ½ t vanilla
    ½ c powdered milk
    1 egg yolk
Place in freezer for about 15 minutes, then transfer to fridge till ready to serve. Stir before using.
Yield: 1 cup

WHIPPED CANNED MILK

To use as whipped cream in a recipe, chill evaporated milk in a bowl in the freezer till ice crystals form around edges of milk. Also chill beaters, either hand or electric.
Whip till stiff:
    ¾ c canned evaporated milk.

Variation: for desserts, chill and whip as above. Add and continue beating till milk is stiff: 1 T lemon juice. Blend in 2 T honey and ½ t vanilla. This will hold up for about an hour if refrigerated.
Yield: about 1½ cups

Variation: chill in bowl as above, whip: ½ c evaporated milk. Add and continue beating: 4 T lemon juice, 4 T powdered milk, 4 T sugar, 1 t vanilla and ¼ t almond extract. Serve over fresh fruit cup.
Yield: about 1½ cups

CAROB DESSERT SAUCE

Blend in blender:
    1 c water
    1 T dark brown sugar
    1 c carob powder
Pour into saucepan and cook gently, stirring constantly to eliminate the raw taste of carob. Serve over any vanilla pudding or frozen dessert. Also mix with milk for "chocolate" milk.
Yield: 1½ cups

FRESH FRUIT TOPPING

In blender:
    1 orange, peeled, seeded and cut in quarters
Add one-third of the total each time:
    5 medium apples, cored and sliced
    1 c cranberries, fresh or frozen
Add and blend till smooth:
    2 T honey
    ½ t cardamom
    ½ t cinnamon (optional)
Use as topping for yogurt, French toast, pancakes, cottage cheese. Or eat as dessert topped with real whipped cream or other topping. Cover and store in fridge.
Yield: 8 servings

DESSERT TOPPINGS

1. 1 c wheat germ, sweetened with ¼ c honey and toasted in oven on large cookie sheet. Mix with 2 T ground almonds or walnuts if desired.
Yield: 1¼ cups
2. Vanilla sauce: Mix in blender: 2 c milk, 4 T honey, 3 t cornstarch, 2 eggs. Cook till mixture coats spoon, and flavor with 1 t vanilla, 1½ t lemon extract or ½ t almond extract.
Yield: 2½ cups
3. Carob sauce: Blend in blender: ¼ c honey or dark brown sugar, 1 c milk, 2 T powdered carob, 2 T powdered milk. Cook till slightly thick. Cool. If sauce separates, stir well.
Yield: 1½ cups

CONFECTIONS

Easy, quick candies to prepare, and all right for the children to eat.

PEANUTTY POPCORN

Preheat oven to 350 F. Mix together:
    3 quarts popped popcorn
    1 c toasted peanuts
Heat together gently:
    ½ c melted butter
    ½ c honey
Pour the butter mixture over the popcorn mixture. Mix well. Spread on a cookie sheet in a thin layer. Bake about 10–15 minutes or till crisp. Break into serving-size pieces.
Yield: 14 servings

FUDGIE SESAME

Place in blender:
    1½ c sesame seeds
    ½ c toasted peanuts
    ½ t vanilla
    2 T honey
    ¼ c (½ stick) butter
Blend till smooth. Divide into halves. To 1 half, add 1 T carob. To the other half, add 2 T shredded coconut. Shape into balls. No coating needed. Store in fridge.
Yield: about 30 balls

INEZ'S CAROB BALLS

Mix together, form into balls and roll in coconut:
    ½ c honey
    ½ c sesame seeds
    ½ c sunflower seeds
        ground in blender
    ½ c fresh ground wholewheat
        flour or wheat germ
    ½ c carob
    ½ c chopped walnuts
    1 t vanilla
Store in fridge.
Yield: about 40 balls

NUTTY OATS

Mix together:

¼ c peanut butter
½ c honey
¼ c butter
Add, mix well, and form into roll 2″ thick:
1 beaten egg
½ t vanilla
1 t orange extract
1 c oatmeal
1 c wholewheat flour
½ c chopped nuts

Wrap roll in waxed paper and refrigerate overnight. Cut in ⅛″ slices, bake on ungreased cookie sheet at 350 F for 8 to 10 minutes. Remove from pan immediately and cool on rack.
Yield: about 40 cookies

SUPER SOYBEANS

Soak in fridge overnight:
¼ c dry soybeans
1 c cold water
Drain, dry on paper towels, and roast at 200 F for 2 hours. Add:
1 T butter
Place under broiler and toast, stirring often till brown.

Or: Add any herb or spice to your taste.
Yield: 4 servings

SPICED NUTS

Combine only till mixed, not foamy:
1 egg white
2 T honey
Add and stir till well coated:
½ t salt
½ t ginger
½ t cinnamon
¼ t nutmeg
¼ t powdered cloves
2 c pecan or walnut halves
Spread in buttered pan and sprinkle with:
date sugar
Bake at 300 F for 30 minutes. Remove from oven and cool slightly. Spread on waxed paper, separating nuts from each other.
Yield: 8 servings

SESAME SEEDS PLUS

Mix in a processor (steel blade) until a mass forms:

1 c sesame seeds
Add:
1 t vanilla
Add through chute:
honey, until the mixture is the consistency of bread dough
Pinch off pieces, roll into balls and press a nut half into the top of each.
Yield: 16 balls

CAROB SAUCE

To make carob sauce, mix together the first 8 ingredients in the next recipe (Carob Clusters). Use the sauce for bread puddings, cake, homemade ice cream, and other desserts.
Yield: 1½ cups

CAROB CLUSTERS

Set oven at 250 F. Mix well in blender:
½ c hot water
¼ c butter (½ stick)
Add and blend well:
¼ c honey or dark brown sugar
¼ c carob powder
¼ c soy powder
1 t vanilla
½ T lecithin granules
⅛ t salt
Turn into bowl and add:
½ to ¾ c non-instant powdered milk
Stir until well mixed. Add one or more of the following:
½ c shelled toasted peanuts
½ c raisins
½ c toasted almonds
½ c toasted cashews
¾ c shredded fresh coconut
Mix well and drop by spoonfuls on foil-lined cookie sheet (dull side of foil next to food). Bake for 10 to 12 minutes.

If the mixture is rather soft, the candies will be chewy. If stiff, the candies will be hard like cookies. All of them will become more firm after they've stood a while, even if they are not cooked at all. Experiment with the consistency your family prefers. They taste good and are healthful snacks.
Yield: 5 dozen

15

A LITTLE OF EVERYTHING

SNACKS

Snacks are universally accepted, and we accept them, too. But our nutritious snacks build health. In fact, we suggest that everybody eat six small meals a day—three main meals at the usual times, and three mid-meals or snacks.

Snacks may be small amounts of protein and fruit. Good snack proteins are natural light colored cheeses, whole grain crackers, nuts, seeds, yogurt, homemade health cookies, cake, pie, ice cream, candy or almost any natural food, especially if it is enriched with non-instant powdered milk or soy powder. If you like desserts, don't eat them with meals; save them for mid-meal snacks. They're all high protein, and you can often choose snacks made with fruit and protein both. See the dessert section for ideas (pp. 109–124).

Snacks should be just snacks—not big meals. Part of this entire idea of nutrition is not to eat too much at one time because that overloads the digestive system, and we can't assimilate the food. Therefore, our main meals are small so we can later eat a snack between meals and at bedtime. As we've said, every snack should be high protein. Therefore, if we do eat fresh raw fruit as a snack, we should eat a few almonds and a few sips of milk with our apple—or half an apple, or even a quarter of an apple. "Bread" no longer means a "piece" of bread—it may mean a quarter of a piece—just a few bites to take the edge off your hunger and to keep the blood sugar up and keep you energetic till lunch or supper time. Add a few nuts or a glaze of peanut butter to any bread to increase the protein value.

Snacks are probably thought of as something to carry in your hand while eating. It would also be nice, however, to make snack time a relaxing time to sit down with a small serving of yogurt and fruit, cottage cheese and a cookie, or cracker and peanut butter. Have the girls over for a gab fest sparked with good nutrition—a sliver of cheese cake with fresh fruit or one of the gelatin desserts made with milk and fruit.

Let's consider some of both kinds of snacks—the carrying kind and the relaxing kind. Popcorn comes to mind first. It's easy to carry or to sit and eat. Make a small amount—it's hard to stop eating popcorn. And, after all, there's another meal coming.

Seeds and nuts are best eaten raw, except for peanuts. We always cook peanuts and all other legumes. But if your family doesn't go for raw seeds and nuts, toast some and mix with untoasted—you'll have the food value of the raw and the taste of the toasted. These are easy to carry in purse or pocket in small plastic bags. Don't go overboard on these high-fat foods, but don't eliminate them from a weight-reducing diet, because we need a little fat throughout the day for energy.

Best of the seeds are sunflower, sesame and pumpkin. Chia, caraway, poppy and many others can be eaten, but usually these are used as garnish on breads or in salads. Don't forget coconuts. Nut butters go right along with other snacks. They can be made with peanuts as we're well used to; but also, they're good when made from almonds, sesame seeds, cashews, filberts, pine nuts, walnuts and Brazil nuts. Most of these have enough oil without adding any.

In making nut butter, grind the peanuts in a

meat grinder with the "worm feed crusher" for oily substances. Grind a few peanuts at a time, toasted and unsalted. Then add the amount of butter that will make the texture you like. Add as little salt as your taste will allow.

All nuts can also be blended to powder in the blender. Then if needed, add butter and a little salt. Try mixing the kinds of nuts and seeds, as three part peanuts, one part sunflower seeds, and a little butter and salt. Here's another: two parts any nuts, one part sunflower seeds, one part sesame seeds, and a little butter and honey. The kids can eat these—all they want.

Frozen bananas make good snacks in many different ways. First, just plain frozen. Peel, freeze on a tray and eat. They taste like banana ice cream. Or peel, roll in a mixture of carob powder and water. Add water to the powder until it's thick but not too thick. After coating the banana, roll in grated coconut or chopped toasted peanuts. Freeze in plastic bags.

TRAIL MIX

Combine all ingredients and serve as snacks:
 ¾ c peanuts, roasted
 1 c cashews, raw or roasted
 1 c coconut shreds
 1 c carob chips
 1 c sunflower seeds, roasted
 1 c raisins
 pinch salt (optional)
Yield: 5¾ cups

CORNMEAL CRACKERS

Combine the following ingredients:
 1 c yellow cornmeal
 1 T butter
 ¼ c sesame seeds
 ½ t sea salt
 ⅞ c boiling water
Drop by tablespoons on buttered baking sheet. Spread in 3 or 4 inch rounds. Bake at 400 F till golden.
Yield: 10 crackers

WHEAT GERM STICKS

There are many good recipes for crackers, all of which make good snacks. I call this one "the greatest."

Mix in small bowl of mixer:
 1¼ c milk
 1 T honey
 ½ c butter
Add and mix for two minutes:
 2 c wholewheat flour
 1 t salt
 2 c wheat germ (or half bran)
Shape into a little loaf about 1″ high, 3″ wide and 8″ long. Freeze. Slice and bake at 325 F about 20 minutes or till brown.
Yield: 24 sticks

YOGURT DIP

Blend to a paste in blender:
 6 walnut halves
 1 T butter
 1 clove garlic (optional)
Stir the blender mix into the following ingredients, chill and serve:
 1 cup yogurt
 ½ t lemon juice or vinegar
 ¼ c finely diced peeled cucumber
Serve with whole grain crackers.
Yield: 1¼ cups

TOFU FOR YOU

Mix all ingredients in blender and serve as a spread or dip or on lettuce leaves:
 1 c tofu
 1 T finely chopped scallion
 2 hard-boiled eggs, mashed
 ¼ c chopped green pepper
 sea salt to taste
Yield:1½ cups

CARROT NUT SPREAD

Blend all ingredients in blender. Moisten with favorite dressing:
 1 c carrots
 1 t lemon juice
 1 c pecans
 1 sprig dill
Yield: 2 cups

CARROT YOGURT COMBO

Set oven to 350 F. Mix well in bowl:

2 beaten eggs
½ c butter melted in pan you'll bake in
½ c honey
¼ c yogurt
Add to egg mixture:
1¾ c wholewheat flour
¼ c soy flour
2 t baking powder
¼ t salt
1½ t cinnamon
Stir in and mix well:
1 c chopped nuts
1 c pitted, chopped dried fruit
1 c grated carrots
Spread in buttered 9″ square pan. Bake 45 minutes. Cut in squares.
Yield: 16 squares

BETTER THAN RAW NUTS

Since raw nuts (except peanuts) have more food value than toasted, we can have the flavor of the toasted and the food value of the raw by preparing nuts and seeds the following way.

Place on cookie sheet:
⅓ of the nuts and seeds to be processed
Bake at 300 F until barely golden brown. Pour at once into a container with a tight-fitting lid. Add the rest of the nuts and seeds, cover the container and shake to mix well. Let stand a few hours, then store in fridge. All the nuts and seeds will taste toasted.

We mentioned peanuts. Never eat peanuts raw—they destroy an enzyme, they may cause goiter and they interfere with digestion.

ENTICING CHILDREN TO EAT

One of the hardest parts of this program is enticing children to eat natural food when they've been brought up on the average American diet of junk food. The older they are, and the longer they've been eating junk, the harder it is to get them to change.

Therefore, if your children are little, and they eat all their meals at home, you've got it made. They'll eat what you buy and prepare.

If they're older, you may have to use your wiles. Here are three methods that have worked for some of my students.

One family of three—mother, father and seven-year-old son—sat down together and discussed Johnny's frequent colds and his not being able to play games at school as being caused by the poor food he was eating. Then they all took turns throwing away some of the junk foods. Next, they all went to the health food store and each one chose something special to be in their new diet—grains, beans, nuts, seeds, dried fruit. Since the whole family decided together, Johnny was enthusiastic about the new diet.

Another family called junk food "poison" in a tone of voice filled with such loathing that the eight-year-old daughter didn't even want to eat it.

Still another mother gave her daughter a $1.00 a week allowance. When Susie begged for a soft drink or candy bar, she was allowed to have it if she bought it out of her allowance. At the high price of such non-foods, Susie very seldom bought any because she was always saving for a doll or some other special gift.

Most important, though, is preparing foods that will build health and satisfy the sweet tooth as well. Any dessert in this book does both. Granola with raisins or carob chips also does both. There are many other special items: Jump-on crackers, frozen bananas with carob coating and toasted peanuts, bars of all kinds, peanut butter and non-instant powdered milk balls rolled in coconut or carob powder.

Don't forget the special drinks—milk and nut milks flavored with carob or fruit, fruit puree with crushed ice or with frozen milk cubes, or frozen fruit blended to a slush with milk.

There's such a variety, it seems impossible that anyone could get tired of the choices. When the children get to be old enough to help make their treats, they'll probably find specialties they become famous for—at least among family members.

PEANUT BUTTER LOG

Very few children of any age would turn down this old favorite—peanut butter—when perked up in this way.

Mix all ingredients together:
  1 c crunchy peanut butter
  ½ c raw honey
  1 to 1½ c non-instant dry milk
  1 t pure vanilla
  ½ c wheat germ
  dash of salt (optional)
Knead until well blended. Form into a log and roll in chopped toasted peanuts or wheat germ. Store in refrigerator. Freezes well for serving later.

GINGERBREAD FIGURES

Set oven at 350 F. Blend together:
  ¼ c butter
  ¼ c unsulphured molasses, warmed
  ¼ c water
Add and mix well:
  1 c wholewheat pastry flour
  ½ t sea salt
  ½ t ginger
  ¼ t nutmeg
Chill for a few hours, pat out ⅜ inch thick and cut into shapes. Let your children draw designs with a toothpick. Bake for 6 to 8 minutes.

FATS AND OILS

Fats and oils are needed in the diet, but the average American eats 45 percent of his calories as fat, and that's too much. Current thinking suggests from 10 to 20 percent of calories as fat. Nutritionists don't agree as to how much should be saturated and how much unsaturated. Some say half and half; some say 80 percent saturated and 20 percent unsaturated.

The most recent figures available show that unsaturated vegetable fat is now up from 4 to 16 percent of the diet (Olson, 1978). Now polyunsaturated fats are being labeled as causing cancer; they seem to be responsible for the carcinogens in dietary fats (Olson, 1978). Of course, a small amount of linoleic acid, the one essential fatty acid that we have to eat because the body can't make it, is essential. "Essential" means we'll die without it. The best sources of linoleic acid are nuts and seeds. These foods also furnish vitamins, minerals and proteins.

After thirty years of being told not to eat cholesterol and to eat large amounts of polyunsaturated fat, we now have plenty of evidence that we've been told wrong (Corday, 1980). Recent research shows that in a five year study of 8,341 patients who had had one or more heart attacks, more of the patients taking cholesterol-lowering drugs and vegetable oils died than those not taking the drugs and oils. Corday says, "People are so different that it is irresponsible to make blanket claims such as are being made to the general public now to reduce the amount of eggs and butter in the diet and to eat margarine, hard white shortening and vegetable oil." The Food and Nutrition Board of the National Research Council of the National Academy of Sciences announced that the "fear of cholesterol in the diet now seems to be greatly overrated." The statement continues, "The medical profession must realize that cholesterol, which has been widely reported as being bad for health, is actually needed to perform many vital functions in the human body." From 1,000 to 2,000 mg of cholesterol is manufactured in the body every day. It makes up 5–10 percent of brain tissue, part of the sex and adrenal glands and part of the membrane of every cell in the body.

Most of the cholesterol the body uses is made from products other than cholesterol, so the conclusion of the Board was that it could not make any specific recommendations about dietary cholesterol for healthy persons.

Dr. Linus Pauling (*Rejuvenation*, 1981) says, "The warning against eggs because of their high content of cholesterol has been made without scientific justification. I believe that eggs are an excellent food, and one egg a day, or even more, usually leads to an improvement in health rather than to damage."

Also, saturated fat is no longer considered the bugaboo it was for the last twenty or thirty years. We must have fat for energy. Some of the best fats are butter, cream, and eggs—all highly saturated and all healthful in moderation. The hard white saturated fat which is marbled through muscle meats (steaks, roasts, chops and hamburger) seems to be the fat to avoid because the poisons that the animal takes into its system in air, feed and water are detoxified by the liver and stored in fat cells. Even if we trim off all visible fat, the meat is still 20 to 50 percent fat. The people who eat large amounts of such fat are often the people who have heart disease and cancer.

One of the worst kinds of oil or fat we can eat is hydrogenated oil, which is hardened vegetable oil. Hydrogen is bubbled through the oil, which becomes solid at room temperature. This is how margarine and hard white shortening are made. Hard margarine is as saturated as butter. Soft margarine is 60–80 percent saturated fat. Both are man-made, not natural fats. A "low-calorie spread" is a mixture of water and hard margarine, which is not good, either. These fats don't get rancid, but they are so altered by the hydrogenation process that the essential fatty acids are destroyed or changed into abnormal fatty acids that our bodies can't use. When we eat these man-made fats, what happens to them? They stack up in our cells as garbage, and the cells can't function well. Investigators say that if we don't die of a killer disease, the garbage that accumulates in the cells will gradually kill us (Hunter, 1971).

Most bottled vegetable oils in supermarkets have been so refined that much of their value has been destroyed. The oil is treated with caustic soda, lye or other strong alkalis, then steamed or mixed with water to remove other impurities. Then it is filtered, bleached and deodorized at a high temperature. It is distilled with steam for up to twelve hours, then filtered again. Finally the oil is bottled as a clear, odorless product with very little nutritional value. It contains chemical antioxidants that keep the oil from spoiling and that may cause cancer (Hunter, 1971).

Cold-pressed oils are usually misnamed. "Cold pressed" can apply only to sesame and olive oils. Sesame oil is said to be the slowest of all vegetable oils to deteriorate, but unrefined sesame oil is very strong-flavored, and most people don't like it in salad dressing. Since olive oil is a monounsaturated fat, rather than a polyunsaturated fat, it doesn't have the one essential fatty acid that the body can't manufacture and that we have to eat. The so-called cold-pressed oils are colder than some others, but they're still heated so hot that they're not healthful.

Studies show that rabbits that ate oil heated to 375 to 400 degrees F had increased incidence of heart disease. In monkeys, peanut oil from the supermarket caused more advanced heart disease than butter. In human development, such oils have been used only a short time, comparatively, and man hasn't had time to adapt to the new processed, heated oils (Ballentine, 1978).

Safflower oil is said to be the most irritating oil because it is the most unsaturated, and therefore can become rancid most easily (Ballentine, 1978). Vitamins E and C help as antioxidants, that is as protectors against rancidity from oxygen, but it is not known if they help enough; and obviously, many people don't get enough vitamin E and C. Unrefined peanut oil is considered good for cooking because when it's heated, it doesn't "gum up" utensils as corn oil does. But we need to reduce intake of all vegetable oils. Coconut and palm oil may be better.

Recent research has shown that consuming polyunsaturated fats does not reduce the risk of heart attack. But Americans who watch TV usually think it does. The FDA says it is illegal for manufacturers to claim that polyunsaturated fats help prevent heart attacks, but when a commercial says "rich in polyunsaturates," people relate it to lessened chance of heart attacks (Ballentine, 1978). Also, physicians noted that their patients with malignant melanomas (highly malignant form of skin cancer) had recently switched to using large amounts of vegetable oils instead of butter (Ballentine, 1978).

Even oil from health food stores is not recommended. Unrefined oil becomes rancid in two days after we take the top off and the oil is exposed to oxygen. Cold-pressed oils are not recommended either. When either type of oil is heated to high temperatures, the structure of the oil molecules is changed, and it doesn't fit the chemistry of our cells. Oils heated to temperatures over 250 F are less digestible then unheated oils. The higher the temperature and the oftener they're heated, the more toxic they get. The oils can form new harmful compounds such as benzene.

Clarified butter is highly recommended. It is said to retard the deterioration of food and to even increase the nutritional value. There are no laboratory studies to support this, but it is known that clarified butter will keep for long periods without refrigeration and will not deteriorate. It has almost all the nutritional value of butter. This butter will not scorch or turn black. People in other parts of the world have used this kind of butter for centuries, especially in France and India (Ballentine, 1978).

To make clarified butter, heat ½ pound of butter in a moderate skillet. The milk solids rise to the top as foam. Skim that off and throw it away. Use the clear yellow oil for occasional frying.

Butter is a natural fat that melts at room temperature, and is a good fat for eating and cooking. We should use it moderately, as we use all fats. The best butter is labeled "made from sweet cream." Other butters are made from stale or soured milk or cream with a lot of salt added to stop the growth of mold, and an alkaline salt added to make the first salt taste less salty (Goldbeck, 1973). We should buy only U.S. Grade AA or U.S. 93 Score. Others can have off flavors from aging. Best is unsalted. Any butter may have artificial colors. Some supermarkets list on the label "colored seasonally," which means that when the grass eaten by the cows isn't green enough to make yellow butter, color is added.

Butter can be stored by the market for months. If you get a pound that has an off flavor or odor, return it. If you want whipped butter, you can easily whip it in your blender. Add ice water gradually to soft butter till you get the consistency you want. Use butter in cooking. It furnishes energy, but we shouldn't eat too much. "Moderation" is our middle name.

Lecithin is a fat that's important in a health food diet. It is in all grains, nuts and seeds, but it is also used as a food supplement made from soybeans to keep the fat in the blood liquid so it will flow through the blood vessels and not stack up as fatty plaques.

The best lecithin to buy is the granular form. The best granules have a high amount of phosphatidyl choline, which is the form that is most active in keeping the blood and the liver free from fatty deposits. Look on the lecithin label to make sure you get the highest percentage of phosphatidyl choline (PC). PC is such a concentrated form of lecithin that instead of taking 4 to 6 tablespoons of lecithin, you may need only 1 tablespoon or less. Since there is so much less volume, it is much easier to take. Dr. Robert Downs in BESTWAYS (November, 1982) says that it is safe, non-toxic and *most* effective.

Mostly, lecithin helps us utilize other fats. It also helps prevent gallstones (Adams and Murray, 1973). We can add lecithin to any liquid. It makes milk taste like cream. We can add it to juice, soup, gravy or stew. It makes fat disappear, because it emulsifies the fat. That isn't so good with gravy or stew. The fat should be skimmed off so we won't eat it. We can mix lecithin with vegetables before serving, with hamburger, meat loaf and scrambled eggs. The only rule is not to add so much that the taste of the food is changed. One of the reasons why we can eat eggs without fear of cholesterol build up is that lecithin in eggs counteracts the cholesterol in eggs. Also, lecithin along with beans and peas helps lower the incidence of heart attacks (Ballentine, 1978). Nature, again, made a food that's good for us and builds health.

How much total fat should we eat? Many nutritionists suggest that we eat no more than 10 to 20 percent of our calories as fat in order to reverse atherosclerosis. We can take vegetable oils as seeds, beans and grains. We should consume very little cooking or salad oils; save them for an occasional meal at friends' homes or in restaurants. Eat no margarine or vegetable shortening. We can include a little butterfat, but very little meat because even lean meat is 20 percent fat of the worst kind (Ballentine, 1978).

In choosing fats and oils to eat, then, we should eat butter, cream and eggs for animal fats which give us energy, and eat nuts and seeds for vegetable fats. We need very small amounts of vegetable fats—the equivalent of three to six teaspoons of vegetable oil a day. Equivalents of one teaspoon of oil are two teaspoons sesame, sunflower or pumpkin seeds, two walnut halves, four pecan halves, six almonds or twelve peanuts. Eat any one of these servings six times through the day, and the fat will burn fat. Eat all six at one time, and you'll get fat.

Exciting new research on vegetable oils reports on linoleic acid, an essential fatty acid (EFA), which has two major uses in the body: (1) it is part of the covering of every cell in the body, especially the cells in the brain, and (2) it is converted to prostaglandins, which regulate the way each organ works. Linoleic acid must be changed to another form—gamma-linolenic acid. (GLA). Without GLA, people may suffer from edema, asthma, acne, menstrual cramps, hyperactivity, multiple sclerosis and other complaints. To help avoid these ailments, we eat nuts and seeds and we don't eat margarine, hard white shortening and processed oils which block the change of linoleic acid to GLA.

EATING WITH FRIENDS

Some people I counsel say, "I'll never be able to eat with friends—in their homes, at restaurants or cafeterias. How can I entertain friends at my home?"

It's easy.

EATING OUT

All of us get "caught" once in a while and have to eat out. In fact, if we could get in restaurants the good food we're used to at home, we'd like to eat out more often than we do. Let's see what we can do about it.

Mexican restaurants always have avocados. They're excellent food. You may not be able to get fresh avocados, but the frozen ones, already mashed and combined with tomatoes and onions as guacamole, are acceptable. Beans are good food, but beans as well as tortillas may be fried in stale fat; the soft tortillas called suaves may be the best bet. Rice, being a grain, should combine well with beans to make complete protein, but the rice is always white, so it's deficient in B vitamins.

Chinese restaurants will serve you good crisp vegetables. We hope they're steamed instead of stir fried because the stir frying at high temperatures requires too-hot oil. The little bits of meat served are not really enough protein to

count, but maybe you won't be eating there too often.

At other restaurants and cafeterias, roast beef is a good choice if you don't choose it too often. Order baked or broiled fish if it's on the menu. All restaurants usually have fried fish with a thick crust. Just throw away the crust and inside you'll find steamed fish. We don't eat the crust because it's soaked in hot oil that is carcinogenic. This eliminates French fried potatoes and onion rings. If you know anyone who eats a lot of French fries, he may be one of the cancer statistics expected by the year 2050, when it is predicted that one of every two people will have cancer. If calves' liver is on the menu, choose that. Chicken livers may not be good; traces of arsenic have been found in them.

Cafeterias have all their hot foods on steam tables where the nutrients continue to be destroyed as the vegetables and meats sit and wait to be eaten. Much food value stays in the liquid in the pans. Cafeteria bread is usually white or "wheat," which usually doesn't mean whole wheat. It's best to pass up the bread—it's hard to find good bread when eating out.

Canned or frozen peas or orange juice may be listed on restaurant menus as "fresh." Scallops, artificially colored pink, may be substituted for lobster, and other items may not be what you think you're getting (Hunter, 1971).

Many specialties of the house may be frozen items, just like the ones you can buy at your frozen food counter, but you pay several times the price at the restaurant. However, you don't have to cook the food yourself, and you get good service and atmosphere.

My favorite meal at a cafeteria is baked fish. Another good choice is cottage cheese and fruit. Most cafeterias have a choice of fresh fruits—watermelon; cantaloupe; apple, celery, and walnut salad; other fruit salads. Skip the bread there, too; it's almost always white. Cornbread has probably had the germ removed. We should try to get wholewheat muffins or biscuits every time we eat out. Ask for them. If enough people ask, someone may take the hint. Buttermilk is often sold in cafeterias; it fills in the cracks in your stomach if enough else isn't there.

Raw vegetable salads are usually good to eat, unless the only "green" vegetable is iceberg lettuce. Choose dark green leaves for about four times the food value of the white. Beets, carrots, green beans, chickpeas and red beans help make salads healthful. Sad to say, many processed foods and foods in salad bars are preserved with sulfites, which are very widely used. They keep foods from turning dark. Fruits and vegetables dipped in bisulfite look fresh and crisp and won't discolor even when they are stale.

Sulfites are also used on shellfish and fried potatoes and many other foods. When people with asthma or bronchitis eat sulfite-sprayed foods, they may have vomiting, heartburn and indigestion. Usually a mineral called molybdenum can change the damaging sulfites to safe sulfates, but molybdenum is in short supply in the average American diet (Papaioannou and Pfeiffer, 1984).

For dessert, choose cheese; forego gelatin desserts—they're too sweet and gelatin is a poor protein. Baked custard should be a good choice. The pies are lined up in rows of empty calories; skip them altogether.

My favorite meal at a restaurant is baked potato and salad. I forego the entree which is usually a too-big serving of animal protein. Not that the animal protein is so bad, but the servings are so large. Almost everybody else gets up from the table gaseous from eating too much and from drinking water, iced tea or coffee with meals. They can't digest and assimilate all that food, and they're shortening their lives with every such meal.

If you don't mind wasting money, order the full meal and eat half of it. Or, if you're with a good friend or a spouse, one of you order a salad and the other a meal. Divide the main course; you'll each have a salad, and you won't overeat. The waiter won't like it, but it's *your* health.

EATING WITH FRIENDS AT THEIR HOMES

When you go to friends' houses, you'll have to eat. Usually when friends invite you over, they prepare food from scratch, and the meat and vegetables should be good. As for salads, they're usually white head lettuce, but there may be tomatoes and other raw vegetables.

Eat some. Don't feel obliged to eat all the white head lettuce. As for the bread, pass it up. The hostess will probably think you're trying to lose weight. In our culture, if you're dieting to lose weight, you're excused for not eating bread; but if you're trying to improve your health, you're considered a health food nut, and that's inexcusable to the average hostess.

Now comes the dessert. Pass it up completely, if possible. If your hostess has made her specialty, eat a few small bites, rave about it, and say you've eaten so much else you can't hold another bite. How about a doggy bag to take the rest home? You've made a hit with her, and you've saved your health. Now when you get home, you can have one of your wheat-germ cookies that build health with every bite.

ENTERTAINING FRIENDS

That leaves the easiest of all—entertaining friends at home. Search the sections of this book for menus. Prepare some of the following:

roast lean beef
broccoli with cheese sauce, topped with toasted
   almonds
bran muffins

Your guests won't be overloaded; they'll feel satisfied, and they'll enjoy the taste of the food. Here's another quickie menu:

baked fish
small serving sweet potato
romaine salad with dressing

And another:

no-meat loaf with sauce
cauliflower with grated cheese and toasted
   sesame seeds
Celery and carrot sticks with your favorite
   dip

If your guests linger late, serve a sliver of cheesecake or a fresh-fruit gelatin dessert at 9:00 or so.

Your guests will no doubt ask you for recipes, and maybe you'll start others on the road to health via natural foods. What better service could we do for our friends?

BROWN BAG LUNCHES

Brown bagging your lunch will probably be the best way to get something healthful if you work or go to school.

For a high-protein dish—and protein is the first thing we settle on for a meal—here are five choices, one for every day in the week.

If you're still eating meat, make a meat loaf, fortified with extra protein such as eggs, soy powder or powdered milk. Slice and freeze for several weeks of meat loaf sandwiches. Next, cheese—any variety that's natural and light colored (no orange dyes). Wednesday is the day for peanut butter and sprouts, Thursday for tuna fish salad. If the tuna seems too salty, as it does to me, blot it between paper towels or combine it with apple to cut the salty taste. On Friday, you'll welcome egg salad with toasted sesame seeds.

All of these sandwiches will be spread on the good wholegrain bread you make yourself, and garnished with crisp romaine leaves or some other leaf lettuce. For the rest of the meal, eat raw vegetables.

Yogurt or buttermilk and fruit as mid-meals will add more protein to your day. If your office or shop doesn't have a fridge, buy a container that keeps food cold. Some are made like handbags; you put the top in the freezer every night and it keeps the container cool at least till noon the next day.

SANDWICH SUGGESTIONS

1. Nut butter with sliced apple, sliced banana, grated carrots, honey, dried fruit.
2. Mashed cooked soybeans or other beans, mixed with ground sesame seeds, chopped onion (optional), sweet peppers, chopped nuts, minced dried apricots.
3. Chopped nuts mixed with grated carrots, chopped celery, wheat germ, a little milk or yogurt, and 1 teaspoon honey.
4. Chopped hard-boiled eggs mixed with Linda's salad dressing (p. 97), chopped fresh herbs, chives, onion, sweet pepper, relish, olives, sprouts.

5. Dry cottage cheese mixed with chopped fresh vegetables or fruits, seasoned with chopped fresh herbs.
6. Peanut butter sandwich with alfalfa sprouts and romaine lettuce on homemade whole-wheat bread.

OTHER FOODS TO CARRY

Yogurt, with or without fresh fruit (don't buy yogurt with fruit in it—too sweet).

Vegetable sticks to eat with nuts and seeds. Salad dressing not necessary.

Kefir or buttermilk. Fresh fruits in season.

Cookies—any natural food recipe. There are hundreds of excellent recipes, or make up your own. Begin with a muffin recipe and add nuts, powdered seeds, carob chips, coconut, raisins, dried fruit. Pat into a $9 \times 9 \times 1''$ pan. Cut into bars—easy to wrap and carry.

SALT

Use sea salt that comes in large crystals, or vegetable salt. Both are from the health food store, and both are primarily sodium chloride so we don't want to overdo even these kinds of salt. The large crystals of sea salt can be ground to powder in a blender or seed and nut grinder. Keep the ground salt in a jar and add a little to the salt shaker when needed. This kind of salt cakes easily and has to be stirred occasionally. Keep a little brown rice in the salt shaker so the salt won't cake.

COFFEE

Since we're saying, "Don't drink coffee, with caffeine or without," we'd better tell you what it can do to you.

You may not realize it, but you can't coordinate your muscles well if you've had caffeine. Also, your timing can be affected. Real or decaffeinated coffee can make you produce more stomach acid (not the right kind). The body must eliminate the excess acids or we have trouble.

If you'd like to keep the hair on your head,

think twice before drinking coffee. It causes B vitamins to be excreted fast; we may have thin hair or even get bald.

Caffeine can cause brain and spinal cord disturbances. It is definitely habit forming, as I find out every time I counsel coffee drinkers. They always say, "Oh, I don't know how I'll get along without coffee." Most of them say they can't get started in the morning without it.

Some people have irregular heartbeats and feel shaky and lightheaded. Some psychologists may tell you it's your spouse, your job or stress; but give up coffee, and those problems will most likely go away.

Coffee also increases the heart rate and perspiration, and causes insomnia and heart palpitations (Gerson, 1958).

Coffee causes the blood sugar levels to drop. Almost everybody knows how serious that can be. It is said there are 100 symptoms of low blood sugar; many of them pertain to the brain (Cheraskin, 1974).

Some people have anxiety symptoms on even one cup of coffee. Caffeine is also the stimulant in cola drinks, cocoa and chocolate flavored foods, and in tea.

Tea also has tannic acid in it and that can destroy iron in the system. Low iron may mean anemia, and those symptoms are often thought to be signs of old age: depression, confusion, clumsiness, sore tongue and general fatigue. Would you ever have thought that drinking tea could have anything to do with those problems? (*Prevention,* May 1980, p. 82). Tea has only ½ to ¾ the amount of caffeine that coffee has, but on an empty stomach, it's just as bad.

MENUS

Menus are so plentiful and varied that you can come up with hundreds of different ones. Each meal should contain protein, so start with that and build around it.

Any animal protein is complete; that is, it has the eight essential amino acids in it (see Chapter 6, Animal Proteins). "Essential" means we'll die without them; usually we don't fall over dead suddenly (although many people do—of a heart attack). Usually we suffer from fatigue—the first symptom of most degenerative chronic diseases. Then we get infections—flu, colds; then digestive problems—gas, bloating, and too-full feeling after meals, or even diverticulosis; then arthritis, heart disease or cancer. So let's have the essentials every day. Other essentials besides proteins are vitamins, minerals, carbohydrates, fats and water.

But we don't have to eat animal protein to get all the amino acids. We can combine plant proteins. All plant proteins have a deficiency of one or more amino acids. But when we combine them we get complete proteins. So we eat nuts, seeds and grains with legumes (beans, peas and peanuts) or either of those categories with milk or eggs (see pp. 56–57).

None of the plant proteins has vitamin B12, so we should use eggs and dairy products or brewer's yeast for that essential nutrient.

After the protein is decided on for lunch, eat a cooked or raw vegetable or both—nothing canned or frozen—and if you're still hungry, a small amount of whole grains either as cracker, muffin, biscuit, bread, or hot cereal in a bowl. Three to six times a day, eat nuts and seeds in these amounts: 2 teaspoons sesame, sunflower, or pumpkin seeds; 2 walnut halves, 4 pecan halves, 6 almonds, or 12 peanuts (see *A Home Study Course in the New Nutrition*, Lesson 1 for details).

By this time, you should feel satisfied, if you've eaten slowly. And that's important, too. Eat slowly, chew every bite till it's like water. Save whole fruit and a few nuts and seeds for a mid meal snack, with ¼ to ½ glass of milk or yogurt.

This way of eating may be different from what you're used to, but it isn't difficult. Most of the difference is in the shopping. We use almost no processed foods except what we process ourselves.

LABELING

Labeling is a controversial subject. It should be helpful, but often it's confusing. We shouldn't have to read labels very often, however, because we seldom buy products with labels. Our major foods are fresh meat, fish, poultry, eggs and dairy products, grains and legumes, fresh vegetables and fruits, and nuts and seeds. Very few of these foods have labels. We do check the label on cheese—it should say "natural."

EXCHANGES AND HINTS

FLOUR

1 c white flour equals: 1 c finely ground wholewheat flour, ¾ c coarsely ground wholewheat flour, ⅞ c wholewheat pastry flour.

If the recipe calls for several cups of flour, as in bread, any of the following may replace ONE cup of wheat flour: ¾ c buckwheat, ¾ c coarse cornmeal, 1 scant c fine cornmeal, ¾ c rye flour, ¾ c soy flour, 1⅓ c oatmeal.

Use other flours with wheat. Soy and other bean flours can be 20 percent of the total. Allow 10–20 minutes extra cooking time and 25 degrees lower cooking temperature. If using other flour when the recipe calls for wheat, use ¾ c buckwheat, oat, or soy.

SUGAR AND SWEETENERS

1 c white sugar equals ¾ c honey.

Use ¼ less liquid, or add 4 T flour. Lower oven temperature by 25 degrees. Or use 1 c molasses, with ⅓ c less liquid.

OTHERS

1 c white rice = 1 c brown rice.

1 c sour cream = 1 c yogurt, but yogurt tends to liquify easily, so add it when not much stirring is needed.

1 oz. chocolate = 3 T carob plus 1 T water and 1 T butter.

3 T cocoa = 4 T carob plus 1 T butter.

Carob is sweet; the amount of other sweeteners may be reduced.

Instead of gelatin you might use agar-agar sold in bars or flakes at health food stores.

Most health food stores carry baking powder without aluminum compounds.

Thickeners: For 1 T white flour, use ½ t arrowroot, potato flour or tapioca dissolved in cold water.

For one cup bread crumbs, substitute 1 c wholewheat bread crumbs, or 1 c wheat germ and 1 raw egg, or ½ c wheat germ, ½ c soy grits and one egg.

For rolling in bread crumbs, use ¼ c each of cornmeal, soy grits, wheat germ, and wholewheat bread crumbs.

Honey causes cookies to be soft. If the cookie should be crisp, add 4 extra T of flour for each ¾ c honey. Bake at about 25 degrees lower temperature.

Instead of salt (sodium chloride), use the same amount of sea salt, earth salt, vegetable salt or dried kelp. Try herbs for seasoning instead of any salt.

Don't use vanillin—use pure vanilla. Try two parts pure vanilla and one part almond in baked goods.

Keep a "soup pot" in the freezer. A 1½ quart plastic pitcher with a top is my choice. I add any leftovers (which are always in small amounts) while clearing the table. Once a month or so we have soup.

"Frizzle" means cook in a moderate skillet with butter. We don't "fry," which means a hot skillet with oil.

Keep spices on one shelf on the inside of the fridge door. It's easy to pick out the one you want, and they keep well.

To use spices herbs, seeds:
1. Grind, crush or chop seeds, nuts and herbs just before adding to food.
2. Steep seasonings by letting the food stand away from heat for a few minutes before being served.
3. Don't cook seasonings at high temperatures.
4. Don't use too much seasoning. You'll ruin the dish.

Here's an easy way to prepare condiments ahead to add to many soups, sauces, vegetables or grain and bean dishes. I use a mixture of olives, pimentos, steamed diced green pepper, (diced onion if you wish) and chopped canned artichoke hearts. Use *your* favorite seasonings.

The trick is to freeze the condiment mixture in a thin sheet so it can be broken apart and used a little at a time without having to thaw the whole mass.

Place the mixture in a plastic bag. *Don't* fasten the bag with a twistem yet. Hold on to the top of the bag with one hand, flatten the contents with the other, press out the air and then fasten the twistem close to the top of the bag. Since the contents are in a thin sheet, you can easily break them apart and use a little at a time.

I grate cheese and freeze it the same way, flattened out in a plastic bag. It keeps well without molding. One of my readers told me another way to keep cheese from molding. Wrap it in cheesecloth or other thin cotton cloth which has been soaked in vinegar. Any size chunks of cheese will keep well. Eventually, the cloth dries out. Just dampen it again and put the wrapped cheese in a plastic bag in the fridge.

You can also freeze the thickeners listed on page 29. Drop one or more of the frozen thickeners into bubbling soup or sauce. It takes a little time to prepare these tricks, but it sure is nice to have them ready when you're in a hurry.

Tamari soy sauce is the best kind of soy sauce. It has no MSG, no sugar, no caramel flavoring.

Place dull side of foil next to food. The shiny side has a coating that can come off on the food.

We used to say, "Don't eat raw egg whites," because avidin in the egg whites destroys biotin (a B vitamin) in the body. Now we learn that that information was based on a study in which rats were fed only large amounts of raw egg whites and no yolks. Yolks have plenty of biotin, so it is safe to eat a raw egg a day, if you eat both white and yolk.

If you want to gain weight, eat a little more fresh cream, butter, nuts and seeds. Eat a lot more complex carbohydrates: whole grains, legumes, vegetables and whole fruits.

16

KITCHEN AIDS

FREEZER

The biggest thing in your kitchen—your freezer—is your biggest helper.

Your freezer makes your new food program easy. Keep foods in bicycle baskets (they're cheaper than freezer baskets).

I have one that I keep all flours and "additives" for baking in. Just one trip from freezer to counter gives me most of my baking ingredients: whole grain flour, soy powder, non-instant powdered milk, bran, wheat germ, and baker's yeast.

Other bicycle baskets hold the following: fish, cooked grains, legumes, nuts, seeds, pureed fruits and fruit juices to be made into jellies through the year. Other shelves hold bags of fruit, tomatoes from the garden and additional sacks of whole grain.

STEAMER

A steamer is the most important cooking utensil in my kitchen. I use mine daily, so I let it sit on the stove all the time. We eat steamed vegetables at least once a day, and I cook grains in it, warm up leftovers and thaw frozen foods. The steamer should have no holes in the bottom, because moisture from the vegetables will fall in the water below, and nutrients will be lost. You can save the water for soup, but it will lose nutrients. It's best to consume any liquid that condenses from the vegetables immediately.

The best steamer is like a wide, shallow double boiler, with steam holes around the top.

A steamer can hold servings of one or more vegetables plus frozen protein dishes you've prepared ahead. Some of the combinations are

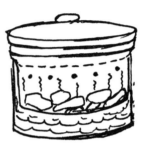

cabbage and/or carrots, grated fine if you're in a hurry to serve the meal, with frozen turkey or salmon loaf. For vegetable stew, cut six or eight vegetables, including potatoes, in chunks. After they're steamed, there will be two or three teaspoons of liquid from the vegetables, with lots of vitamins and minerals in it. Pour the liquid in the serving dish so everybody will get his share. The protein dish this time can be brown rice and red beans. Leave both the rice and the beans in their freezer containers to keep the bean juice separated from the rice, if you wish. There's still plenty of room for the vegetables.

I go in the kitchen 30 minutes before a meal, drink my water and load the steamer. I set the burner to high, set the timer for about 3 minutes, then reduce heat to low—not simmer, that's too low. Then I set the timer for 8 to 20 minutes, and when it calls me back, supper is ready. The food doesn't have to be stirred, and it can't burn. But don't be like me and forget to put water in the lower pan. I burned the bottom out of a pan once.

TIMER

Do you have a good timer? I like the clock timer that tells the time and also has a second hand. Without a timer, I'd burn up a pan every day!

JUICER

I vote for a good juicer—the Champion. Besides being easy to use, with few parts, it releases the juice and the fiber into separate bowls, so you don't have to stop and clean the juicer then start over. The Champion also makes peanut butter and super ice cream. The ice cream you make builds health with its fresh yard eggs, whole milk and very little sweetening.

FOOD PROCESSOR

I'd hate to have to prepare food without a food processor. I held off for a long time before I bought one; I thought it was just one more gadget to find a storage place for. And besides, it would have to be washed.

None of my fears was realized. I leave it on the sink board where it's handy, and much of the time, it needs just a quick rinse when I've shredded vegetables in it. It's worth getting if used for nothing but cabbage slaw or steamed cabbage. It's ideal for carrots. If you have small children or oldsters who can't chew well, use the steel blade and make a fine puree of raw carrots. Chopped carrots are also good, to eat raw or to steam. I like thin sliced celery for salad—delicious with a few nuts and yogurt-base salad dressing.

Baked goods are the easiest ever. Pie crust is quick. Process (steel blade) the dry ingredients, add butter cut in chunks. Process until it's like coarse meal. Add liquid and process till it is sticky crumbs. Pat into pie plate, put another pie plate on top, press down hard while you give the top plate a quick twist, and your crust is thin. It will be crisp and delicious. You can make it faster than I can write this.

You can make muffins this way, too, but don't process more than a few seconds after you add the liquid. It's easy to overdo at that stage. I usually use the blender-bowl method for muffins because I often double the muffin recipes, and that's more than the processor can

hold (see p. 77). If you don't have a processor, put one on your Christmas, Mother's (Father's) Day or birthday list.

BLENDER AND SEED GRINDER

Two other electrical appliances are especially useful: a blender and a seed grinder. I use a blender often to make milk drinks, nut milks, sauces, smoothies, to grind large amounts of nuts and seeds, make apple sauces, combine liquid ingredients for batters . . . ad infinitum. The blender helps make muffins easily (see p. 77). The seed grinder's major use is to grind small amounts of nuts and seeds. Once the seeds are ground, they become rancid quickly, so we grind only as much as we can eat at one time. Seeds and nuts can be ground to a fine powder for people too young or too old to chew well. This gadget will grind as little as one tablespoon of seeds.

COOKWARE

Aluminum pots and pans conduct heat rapidly, the thicker the better. But aluminum pits, and the aluminum is dissolved when acid fruits are stored and when vinegar is used in it. Also, aluminum is discolored when in contact with alkaline foods, hard water or detergent. It is pitted by salty food or water or by copper. Traces of arsenic and fluorides may dissolve in the food. There are many journal reports of danger from aluminum (Hunter, 1971).

Adelle Davis says, however, that aluminum oxide combines with phosphorus and is excreted from the body. Aluminum pots and pans release small amounts of metal into the food, especially if the food is alkaline. Tests show that the aluminum gets into the blood, but it is thought that these amounts are harmless. There is more aluminum in natural foods we eat than we get from pots and pans. However, the forms of aluminum in utensils may be more harmful to the body than the forms in foods (Ballentine, 1978).

Aluminum combines with phosphorus in the body and forms insoluble compounds which pass out of the body with the feces. When this was discovered, doctors began giving people on dialysis machines aluminum to help them get rid of phosphates. Then it was found out that it's possible to get too much aluminum. The controversy continues, but studies show that people with Alzheimer's disease had four times the normal amount of aluminum in their brains. People who take a lot of antacids take in much more aluminum than is received from pots and pans. Schroeder says that antacids and deodorants contain harmful amounts of aluminum, but aluminum cookware and baking powder do not. (Health food store baking powder doesn't have aluminum, but most baking powders contain high percentages of it.) In some cities, aluminum is added to the public water supply to keep it from being murky. It is not known how much aluminum is toxic.

Authorities such as E. J. Underwood and Henry A. Schroeder say that no harmful effects or dangers result from using aluminum cookware or even baking powder that contains aluminum. But it is not recommended that we clean aluminum pans by cooking acid fruits in them. We may clean them by boiling water with 1 T cream of tartar in it, then scrubbing with aluminum cleaner (Pfeiffer, 1975).

If we stay away from deodorants and antacids, use health food store baking powder without aluminum and use our aluminum utensils carefully, we should be safe. The steamer I use so much is aluminum.

Pottery cookware has been used for many years. Modern pots, however, can be glazed with lead or cadmium which contaminates the food.

Other cooking utensils, such as iron or stainless steel, can be used, just so vegetables can be steamed rather than boiled. To steam vegetables, put two tablespoons of water in any heavy pan and when it makes steam, put washed and dried vegetables in. Many people have waterless cookware, and directions come with it.

Stainless steel seems to be good. Some people say the chromium in the steel might combine with the foods, but it probably isn't harmful (Ballentine, 1978). However, Adelle Davis says stainless steel is dangerous because chromium and nickel can leach into the food if the pan has ever been scoured and the finish marred.

Davis suggests stainless steel for soups; aluminum for other foods (Davis, 1947).

Cast iron utensils such as skillets are among the most ideal for cooking because they are usually thick and heavy and they distribute heat more evenly. The food is cooked at a more uniform temperature, so one part of the food won't be underheated while another part is being scorched. These skillets are especially nice for cooking vegetables, because the vegetables are sort of roasted without water, and they can be tenderized yet maintain their shape and flavor (Ballentine, 1978).

The inner surface of the cast iron utensils should be smooth. It is important to take care of them correctly. We have to scrape the food off if any sticks to the pan, but it isn't good to use abrasive cleaners a great deal. After each use, the skillet should be well dried by setting it back on the fire for a moment and then it should be oiled. The surface of the iron develops a smooth tough coating of carbon, and food doesn't easily stick to it. Cast iron pots and pans should never be left in water or with water or acid foods inside. They begin to rust and discolor the food. Even if the iron may be useful to the body, the inner coating of the pan is broken down by the acid foods. Cast iron is considered to be healthful and safe if used carefully.

One of my Chinese nutrition students says that when the pan is first taken off the fire and the contents are removed, the hot pan should be filled with hot water, emptied, and a paper towel swished around in the pan to dry it. The pan is ready to put away. She uses an iron skillet instead of a wok.

Many of my students prefer enameled iron cooking utensils. They're heavy, the tops fit tightly and steam doesn't escape. They say that if the enamel does crack, what's underneath is good old iron, so the crack isn't critical.

Copper pots are dangerous; they shouldn't be used.

Glass, ceramic and glass-ceramic are less subject to the chemical action of foods than metals. They heat slowly and unevenly, but once heated, hold heat well (Hunter, 1971). The problem with ceramic may be that the tops don't fit tightly. Rule them out.

Pressure cookers are all right if the timing is exact (Davis, 1947).

Plastic- or teflon-coated metal is almost an unknown quantity as far as danger or safety is concerned. It is known that plastic can react with food. If temperatures are high, the reaction may be dangerous. Then again, the bad chemicals may be all used up in the first few times the pans are used, and they would be safe after that. This is an experiment whose results we'll await with interest.

Slow cookers are helpful, especially if mother and father both work. Prepare the food the night before, stick it in the fridge, and then slip it into the cooker the next morning. I used to use this utensil often, but now that I'm home most of the day, I use the cooker-steamer almost exclusively. The only kind of slow cooker I recommend has coils in the sides rather than in the bottom. Coils in the bottom make the food boil. I like to use small pans inside the cooker (in my favorite steamer, too) to warm or cook small amounts of food.

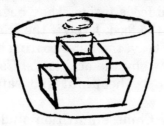

Small aluminum pans, 3×6×2″, are ideal. I recently got some pans 2½ × 4½ × 1½″ deep that go in my steamer. They're nice for liquidy recipes so the liquid won't get in all the food being cooked. They can be stacked at right angles to each other. I can get four of those tiny pans in my steamer. Each pan holds a serving for two people. The small ceramic dishes about 5 × 5 × 1½″ can be used, also. Since none of these small pans has a cover, use foil to keep foods from drying out. These small pans are also good to heat foods in the toaster-oven.

SALAD SPINNER

Another helpful utensil is a salad spinner. The first ones came from France, and they evi-

dently take the place of the young boy who used to fling the greens to dry them outside of restaurants in French villages. The spinners are ideal, especially for large families. With only two in my family, I usually dry my two leaves of romaine and one rib of celery with a turkish towel. We always wash only enough greens for one meal at a time.

MICROWAVE OVENS

Everyone asks me about microwave ovens. Read *The Zapping of America* by Brodeur (W. W. Norton and Co., Inc. NY, 1977). Here are some of his comments:

"The U.S. allowance for microwave radiation is ten milliwatts per square centimeter. But the Russians allow only one-tenth of that amount— one milliwatt per square centimeter." There is a history of cataracts caused by microwave radiation. The brain and the lens of the eye are more susceptible to radiation than are the bones and muscles. Children who look in the door of the oven may have eye injuries because, according to experts, all ovens leak soon after they've been repaired. Also, the one most dangerous source of radiation is that the waves don't cut off as they should when the door is opened.

Ovens are allowed by federal regulation to leak as much as five milliwatts of radiation after purchase. It is not known whether or not this level is safe. The average housewife doesn't have the slightest notion how much or how little radiation her oven is leaking. The manufacturers insist that no harm comes from children looking in the door to watch the food cooking, but no one has any idea what the long-term, low-level effects of microwaves are.

On the jacket of Brodeur's book we read: "Microwave radiation can blind you, alter your behavior, cause genetic damage, even kill you. The risks have been hidden from you by the Pentagon, the State Department, and the electronics industry. With this book, the microwave cover-up is ended."

A government pamphlet says the cook should stay "at least an arm's length away from a microwave oven." Others say the microwaves are zapping the American public. Let's wait to buy one until there's more research done.

TOASTER-OVEN

I talk a lot about a toaster-oven. There are many on the market, and all have almost the same purpose—to make it easy to warm up, toast or even bake foods without heating the big oven.

Some of the toaster-ovens will cook meats from scratch; others will warm foods that have been cooked already. Either kind is good, so when you buy yours, look around at all of them. More and more appliances are coming on the market all the time. We might as well enjoy what is available.

17

QUESTIONS AND ANSWERS

If you were in a nutrition class, you might have questions to ask. Here are some that my students asked in one of my classes.

Q: Can you eat green beans raw?
A: No. Legumes (beans, peas and peanuts) should not be eaten raw. They have three bad reactions on the body: 1. They stick the villi in the intestines together so we can't digest food well; 2. they can cause goiter; 3. they keep the pancreatic enzymes from digesting food. Always cook legumes.

Q: On a vegetarian diet, how do you know when you have a balanced meal?
A: The main problem is getting enough protein and B12. Learn to combine whole grains and legumes for excellent plant protein. At one serving, eat about half as much legumes (beans, peas, peanuts) as grains. Brewer's yeast is a good source of B12, as are all animal proteins. If a vegetarian consumes milk and eggs, he has a much easier way of getting the protein and B12 he needs.

Q: Are meat and fish complete proteins?
A: Yes, they have all eight amino acids in the amounts our bodies need.

Q: How long will raw milk keep?
A: About six days, in my experience, if well refrigerated.

Q: How do you balance proteins in fruits and vegetables?
A: There is so little protein in most of these foods that they are not considered a good source.

Q: Are bulgur and nuts balanced proteins?
A: No. They are in the same category. They should be complemented with legumes.

Q: Are whole grains and lentils balanced?
A: Yes, lentils are legumes, balanced by whole grains.

Q: What about phytates in eating whole grains?
A: It was formerly thought that the phytates in whole grains combined with minerals and eliminated them from the body. Recent research shows that whole grains help the body absorb minerals.

Q: Can you wash vegetables and fruits with soap?
A: Probably the best washing agent is dish detergent. Do rinse well.

Q: Is it all right to buy brown rice at the supermarket?
A: Better to buy it at the health food store.

Q: Do different honeys have different levels of fructose?
A: I don't know. But we don't want to eat much of any kind of honey.

Q: Are there any precautions in buying sesame seeds?
A: The consensus seems to be to buy *hulled* sesame seeds.

Q: Do you like protein powders?
A: No. Rather than eat so much concentrated protein, I think the best proteins as supple-

ments are brewer's yeast and desiccated liver. They contain not only excellent protein, but also all B complex vitamins and minerals.

Q: Where do you get vegetable broth seasoning?
A: At health food stores.

Q: Do you use sea salt?
A: Yes. I use sea salt that comes in large crystals. I grind it in the blender and put rice in the salt shaker to make it free-flowing.

Q: Why do you specify Grayslake gelatin over any other?
A: Other gelatins are less well balanced in amino acids than the health food store kind. Even so, you should add proteins such as cottage cheese, milk, eggs, etc. to Grayslake.

Q: Is sea salt better than sodium chloride?
A: Yes. Sea salt has traces of other minerals.

Q: Is cornstarch any better than arrowroot?
A: Both are acceptable.

Q: What about using baking soda?
A: Soda does destroy some vitamins. But some nutrition-minded cooks say use a minimum of baking soda, and use instead baking powder. Of course, baking powder has soda in it (and acids which help bring about the rising action). We should use no more than 1 teaspoon of baking powder to 1 cup of flour. Eggs will help our heavy wholegrain flours rise. Fold in the egg whites last.

Q: What is a good food yeast?
A: Compare labels on brewer's (food) yeasts at health food stores. They should be balanced with calcium and have substantial amounts of B complex vitamins. You may be surprised at the differences in yeasts. There are several excellent brands at health food stores.

Q: How much low fat milk should we give children?
A: None. We should not fractionate food; that is, take out part of what nature put in. Cream contains five important trace elements, one of which is chromium. Chromium is part of the glucose tolerance factor. Without this factor, we can't tolerate glucose which means that our blood sugar will fluctuate and we may end up with hypoglycemia or diabetes. Feed the children whole milk. Take them off junk food with empty calories, and they won't get fat. Of course, some children drink too much milk. Too much of any one thing is bad, even if it's a good food.

Q: How can you be sure the flour you buy is fresh?
A: By grinding it yourself. If you buy flour, I know of no way to determine its freshness.

Q: Do you have an opinion on microwave ovens?
A: Yes, see p. 140.

Q: How long can you keep powdered milk?
A: The powdered milk from the supermarket will probably keep months on the shelf. The non-instant milk from the health food store I keep in the freezer in my "baking basket." It should keep there indefinitely.

Q: What else do you recommend as food supplements besides calcium?
A: All vitamins and minerals in moderate amounts. Some nutrients may be needed in massive amounts for a short while. You can find charts of recommended amounts of all food supplements in *A Home Study Course in the New Nutrition* (Long, 1983).

Q: Do you think a multi-vitamin is as good as buying vitamins separately?
A: Not usually. It is hard to find a good formula in a multi-vitamin product. I suggest A as beta-carotene, all B complex together, C in powder or crystalline form, D and E by themselves, minerals together, and extras such as lecithin, brewer's yeast, and desiccated liver plus digestive ensymes (hydrochloric acid and pancreatic enzymes). (See lesson 1 of *A Home Study Course in the New Nutrition* [Long, 1983]).

Q: Can you take your calcium all at one time?
A: Minerals and most vitamins should be taken at least twice a day. Oil-soluble vitamins can be taken once. Vitamin C may be needed more than twice, depending on the amount of stress anyone is subjected to.

Q: If you are using brewer's yeast as well as a B-50 tablet, could you be taking too much vitamin B?

A: Highly unlikely. Most adults do well on a B-50 tablet three times a day at main meals. The amount in one heaping tablespoon of yeast is usually no more than 8 milligrams (B 1,2,6). B complex is excreted if not used. Minerals in brewer's yeast may need to be counted in the complete mineral intake, but most people don't get enough minerals. People in excellent health who never suffer from fatigue or stress can try less B complex.

Q: How do you prepare cereal grains for a baby?

A: Don't give babies cereal grains until they are at least six months old. Breastfeed till then, if possible. After six months, cook finely ground unrefined cereals. Mix one part of any cereal with ½ part of noninstant powdered milk from the health food store. Stir slowly into two parts of boiling water. This is a rule of thumb for the amounts of cereal to water. Add ½ teaspoon of brewer's yeast or less, depending on the size serving. Begin with ¼ teaspoon, increasing gradually. Never let cereal take the place of breast milk till age 1 or more.

Q: Is garlic any good for allergies?

A: Garlic is part of the supplements that will bring any ill person to health. Allergies easily clear up on a diet that is as perfect as possible, with moderate amounts of all food supplements; massive amounts of some may be needed temporarily. See *A Home Study Course in the New Nutrition*, Lessons 1 and 4 for details.

Q: Do you recommend using bone meal?

A: No, I recommend calcium and magnesium without phosphorus because most people don't need to add phosphorus to their diets. Natural food enthusiasts get extra phosphorus from whole grains, lecithin, brewer's yeast, and desiccated liver, so they, especially, don't need to add phosphorus.

Q: How do you get extra calcium in the diet?

A: The best source of calcium as a supplement, according to most nationally known nutritionists, is amino acid chelated calcium, combined with half the amount of magnesium, available at all health food stores. Good food sources are cottage cheese, cheddar cheese, and dark green leafy vegetables. Calcium is not well absorbed without milk sugar, vitamin D, and fat (drink whole milk).

Q: What do you need for poor circulation?

A: Vitamin E is a supplement that really helps. If you have high blood pressure, congestive heart failure or diabetes, or if you have ever had rheumatic fever, start slowly with 30 IU a day, go up 30 a month for a year. Then you'll be taking 360 IU a day. Go on up to 600–800 IU. The older you are, the more you take, up to 1200 IU for 70-year-olds.

If you have none of those problems, start with 400 (young women), or 600 (young men). Increase gradually, according to age. Exercise is essential, but this entire diet and food supplement program is aimed at increasing your energy. You'll become so peppy you won't be able to sit around doing nothing. You'll be up and exercising. I get letters from many people who say they are playing tennis, swimming and/or gardening, whereas they had no energy for such activities before they began this diet.

Q: Of the fruit juices, which ones have the least amount of sugar?

A: Grapefruit. However, we get more value from whole fruit. Let's give up fruit juice because of its high content of sugar. There is more to fruit than just juice.

Q: What kind of vegetable oils should be used?

A: None. We need a small amount of polyunsaturated fat, which we get from nuts and seeds. Bottled oil is so processed before it is bottled that it is detrimental to our health. We should use butter for cooking and as a spread on bread.

Q: Is lard a good fat?

A: No. Toxins collect in animal fat. Also, it stays on the shelf unrefrigerated. Let's use butter, cream and eggs as good animal fats, and raw nuts and seeds (always cook peanuts) as vegetable fats.

Q: Are cashews a good source of fats?

A: Yes. All nuts and seeds are good sources,

including coconuts. Too many nuts and seeds will make you fat, but moderate amounts furnish essential fatty acids, energy and incomplete protein, which we combine with beans, peanuts and animal proteins, which furnish all the amino acids.

Q: How much fat is in eggs?

A: There are about 60 calories of fat in egg yolk and about 15 more calories in the white, which is mostly protein. For their excellent food value and high protein content, eggs are among the most healthful foods we can eat. The amount suggested is one or two a day and cook with extra eggs, if we want to make muffins or custards. See *A Home Study Course in the New Nutrition* (Long, 1983) for a discussion of cholesterol, Lesson 3.

Q: What food items should never be bought?

A: White sugar and white flour and any products made from these non-foods. Pork, especially bacon (ham rarely). Canned foods except fish (water packed tuna, salmon, mackerel, sardines). Blot oil from sardines with a paper towel. Frozen foods, convenience foods, coffee, tea, soft drinks with sugar or without, booze, beer, cocoa, fruit juice; processed meats such as hot dogs (except from the health food store), lunch ham and bologna; margarine, hard white shortenings; nuts in cans or jars; tobacco in any form, chocolate, iceberg lettuce (buy dark green leaf lettuce); pastries and desserts; anything fried.

Q: What foods may be bought in supermarkets?

A: Fresh fruits and vegetables, beans and other legumes (lentils, split peas, peanuts in their shells), fresh meat and fish, milk, light-colored natural cheese, cottage cheese, butter, distilled water, popcorn, plain yogurt with live culture (although it's best to make your own).

Q: What foods should be bought in health food stores?

A: All grains if fresh ground and whole. Cheese if you wish, carob, yogurt, vitamins and mineral supplements, non-instant powdered milk, legumes if you wish, eggs and chickens, peanut butter.

Q: What items must be refrigerated?

A: Oils, dairy products, grains cooked or raw, dried fruit ready to eat, nuts, small amounts; dairy products; seeds, small amounts; fruit for short storage; vegetables.

Q: What foods should be kept in the freezer?

A: Grains, cooked or raw; nuts, seeds, fruit purees, raw fruit for long storage, e.g., peaches, foods prepared ahead.

Q: What homemade and bought items should typically be frozen?

A: All breads and cereals cooked and raw—cookies, crackers, muffins, biscuits, granola; fruits for smoothies; foods prepared ahead.

Q: What items can be kept on the kitchen shelf?

A: Dried beans, arrowroot, cornstarch, carob.

Q: Where can you buy good chicken?

A: From a health food store. If your store doesn't stock them, they will be happy to order them for you, but many stores carry them. Look in the freezer.

Q: On your program, how do you get around severe allergy?

A: Allergy is caused by undigested food and other poisons that get into our cells. Of course, our cells are sensitive to poisons. We just have to keep our cells so healthy that the poisons will be destroyed by our body's wonderful immune system. The way to do that is to be sure that every cell gets every nutrient it needs. Then the body repulses the allergens. I have hundreds of letters in my files saying, "no more allergies."

Q: What does acidophilus do for digestion?

A: It keeps the friendly bacteria in the intestines friendly. We have three pounds of microorganisms in our intestines, and if most of them are friendly, they will destroy the poisonous bacteria.

Q: What about a child with a very high IQ but who has a learning disability with several motor-coordination problems?

A: The child should be on a complete natural food diet with moderate amounts of all food supplements and massive amounts of some for a short time. The B complex is especially important, and the B's are not toxic in large amounts. Lecithin, brewer's yeast and desiccated liver are also helpful.

Q: How can you know what supplements everyone needs since every individual is different from all others?

A: Every individual needs all fifty or so nutrients—twenty vitamins, twenty minerals, eight essential amino acids, carbohydrates, fats and water. When I counsel people, I take a medical history, make a diet analysis and put people on a good food and food supplement program and the body will heal itself. So much research has been done that most of man's ailments can be relieved with good nutrition. Sick people are obviously not getting all the needed nutrients. When they are furnished, it is possible to enjoy good health.

Q: When I take 500 milligrams of vitamin B3, I have a severe reaction right away: itching, red face, etc. How come you suggest 750 mgs?

A: The niacin is what causes the reactions. Niacinamide, another form of vitamin B3, does not.

Q: Can you take too much lecithin or vitamin B complex and get an overdose?

A: Yes, we can take too much of anything, but it is highly unlikely. I recommend from one teaspoon to two tablespoons of lecithin, depending on the severity of heart disease or other ailment. I suggest about 50 mgs of vitamin B1, B2 and B6 with three main meals a day, with about five times that much niacinamide and pantothenic acid. It would be highly unlikely that this amount would be too much for an adult unless he had severe digestive problems. If so, grind up the hard tablets (not the gelatine perles or digestive enzymes), and take the powders in small amounts, increasing gradually.

Q: How many mgs of L-glutamine are recommended for small and older children?

A: The adult dosage suggested by Passwater is from two to four 500-mg tablets divided through the day. Thirteen-year-olds take the adult dose. Children from six to twelve take half that much, and from one to six one-fourth that amount.

Q: What is a good source of amino acids for children?

A: There are many new amino acid products coming on the market now. Children can take a percentage of the adult dose which is suggested at 1,500 to 3,000 mgs three times a day depending on their condition. See percentages for children in previous answer.

REFERENCES

Adams, R., and Murray, F.; 1973; *The Good Seeds, the Rich Grains, the Hardy Nuts for a Healthier, Happier Life:* New York; Larchmont Books.

American Laboratory; 1979; *Heated Oils*; September issue.

Ballentine, R.; 1978; *Diet and Nutrition*; Honesdale, PA; The Himalayan Institute.

Cheraskin, E., Ringsdorf, W.M., and Brecher, A.; 1974; *Psychodietetics*; New York; Bantam Books.

Clayson, D.B.; 1975; "Nutrition and Experimental Carcinogens: A Review"; *Cancer Res.* 35:3292–3300.

Corday, Elliott; 1980; *Nutrition Today*; July–August.

Davis, A.; 1947; *Let's Cook It Right*; New York; Harcourt, Brace & World.

Davis, A.; 1965; *Let's Get Well*; New York; Signet.

Downs, R., with van Baak, A.; 1982; "Phosphatidyl Choline: Sensational New Supplement for Circulatory and Nervous Systems"; *Bestways*; November.

Gerson, Max; 1977; *A Cancer Therapy*, 3rd Edition; Del Mar, CA; Totality.

Goldbeck, N. and D.; 1973; *The Supermarket Handbook*; New York; Signet.

Guyton, A.C.; 1976; *Textbook of Medical Physiology*; Philadelphia; W.B. Saunders; pp. 77–81.

Haenszel, W. et al.; 1973; "Large Bowel Cancer in Hawaiian Japanese"; *J. Nat. Cancer Inst.* 51:1765–1769.

Houston *Chronicle*; 1976; Sec. 5; p. 1, July 29.

Hunter, B.T.; 1961; *The Natural Foods Cookbook*; New York; Pyramid.

Hunter, B.T.; 1971; *Consumer Beware!*; New York; Bantam.

Hunter, B.T.; 1980; *Fumigants and Solvents in Food Processing*; Journal of Applied Nutrition, 32(1): 244–257.

Issels, J.; 1975; *Cancer, A Second Opinion*; London; Hodder and Stoughton.

Jansson, B.; 1976: "Cancer Rates—Functions of Carcinogens and Anticarcinogens"; Proc. Conf. Env. Health, Alta, Utah, July 5–9.

Livingston-Wheeler, V., and Addeo, E.G.; 1984: *The Conquest of Cancer: Vaccines and Diet*; New York; Franklin Watts.

Long, R.Y.; 1983; *A Home Study Course in the New Nutrition*; Houston; Nutrition Education Association, Inc.

Nichols, J.; 1972; *Please, Doctor, Do Something*; Atlanta, TX; Natural Food Associates.

Nusz, Frieda; 1972; *The Natural Foods Blender Cookbook*; Keats; New Canaan, CT.

Nutrition Almanac; 1975; New York; McGraw Hill.

Omohundro, D.D.; 1979; "Let Them Eat Bread"; *Consumer's Digest*; September–October; pp. 22–25.

Papaioannou, R. and Pfeiffer, C.C.; 1984: Sulfite Sensitivity—Unrecognized Threat: Is Molybdenum Deficiency the Cause? *Journal of Orthomolecular Psychiatry*, 13(2): 105–110.

Passwater, R.A.; 1976; *Supernutrition*; New York; Pocket.

Pauling, L.; Sugar: "Sweet and Dangerous"; *Executive Health*; Vol. 9, No. 1.

Pauling, Linus; 1981; Introduction to "You Need Never Grow Old"; *Rejuvenation* 9:3–55; September.

Pfeiffer, Carl C.; 1975; *Mental and Elemental Nutrients*; New Canaan, CT; Keats Publishing, Inc.

Rinse, Jacobus; 1973; *American Laboratory*; July.

Shaw, L.; 1980; "Tired? Think About Iron;" *Prevention*; May; p. 82–84.

Shennan, D.H., and Bishop, O.S.; 1976; "Diet and Mortality from Malignant Diseases in 32 Countries"; *Nutr. Abstrs. & Revs.*, 46:268.

Spiro, H.M.; 1976; "Visceral Viewpoints"; *Journal of Applied Nutrition* 28(1):74.

Swartz, June; 1978; *Ed's Farmers Market*; Houston, TX; August 8.

Walczak, M. (Ed.); 1977; *Nutrition Applied Personally*; LaHabra, CA; International College of Applied Nutrition.

Wheedon, J.; 1976; Lecture, University of Texas School of Public Health; Houston.

Williams, R.J.; 1971; *Nutrition Against Disease*; New York; Pitman.

Williams, R.J.; 1973; *Proc. Natl. Aca. Sci.* 70:710–713.

Wynder, E.L., and Bross, I.J.; 1961; "A Study of Etiological Factors in Cancer of the Esophagus"; *Cancer*, 14; 389–413.

Yunis, E.J., and Greenberg, L.J.; 1974; Immunopathology of Aging; *Fed. Proc.* 33: 2017–2019.

SUBJECT INDEX

RECIPE INDEX